I0791774

UPDATING YOGA

A LOOK AT SHASHI YOGA

EARL DICKEY

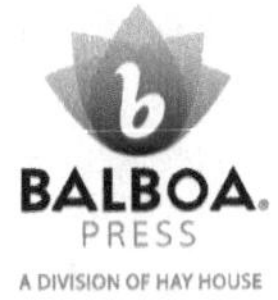

BALBOA.
PRESS

A DIVISION OF HAY HOUSE

Balboa Press books may be ordered through booksellers or by contacting:

Balboa Press
A Division of Hay House
1663 Liberty Drive
Bloomington, IN 47403
www.balboapress.com
1 (877) 407-4847

Print information available on the last page.

ISBN: 978-1-9822-3177-4 (sc)
ISBN: 978-1-9822-3178-1 (hc)
ISBN: 978-1-9822-3182-8 (e)

Library of Congress Control Number: 2019910100

Balboa Press rev. date: 07/31/2019

DEDICATION

To the human body

Salute

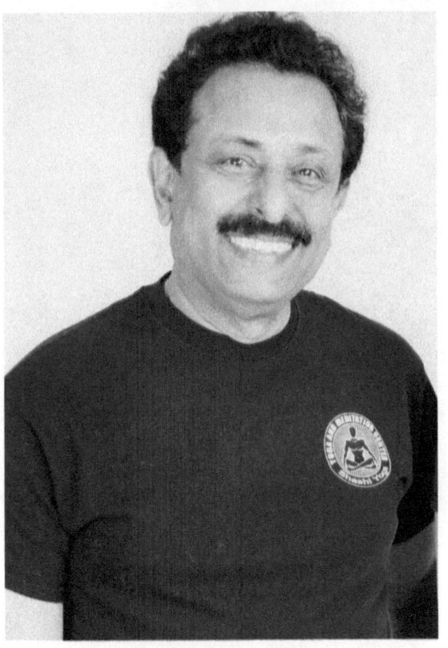

Shashi Pottahil

To Shashi Pottahill & Shashi Yoga, on the approaching 20th Anniversary of his Yoga and Meditation Center.

CONTENTS

ACKNOWLEDGEMENT

To Shashi Pottahil, his secretary Yumi and the many
Yoga Students that encouraged me to write this book.
Also my thanks to BalboaPress Zoe Badger and Dee Garner.
A special thank you to Mel Podell for his encouragement.
And special thank you to Louise, my fiancé,
friend, consultant, and sounding board.

ABOUT THE AUTHOR

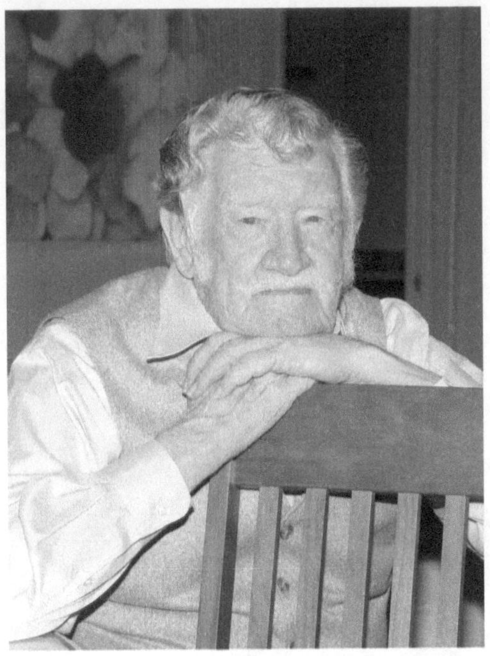

Earl Dickey was born and raised in San Diego. A life long student of religions, yoga and metaphysics. Earl is a Vietnam era veteran, spent six years as a Buddhist monk and was given a name Kandanya. The first student of the Buddha. Earl lives in San Diego California with his fiance Louise.

Mother Yoga & Father Science

My Dear Mother Yoga, from the Valley of Sweetness, in the County of Caring, you were born. It was there in a Lotus Pond, from its most beautiful flower, that you did emerge.

The ponds' flower and you, were the talk of the town. Of how you shine with such brilliance, as no one has seen. While the sound of your voice, is far above a Musicians' dreams.

High on a mountain, your father is so pleased, he danced and danced, as you gave life to his dream. Even the atoms within us continue to dance, for you give us all hope and a wonderful chance.

You married early a farmer named Science. Father Science toiled long hours in the fields of Knowledge. In the Orchards of Academia he picked the sweetest of the fruits of learning.

Although your family is large. You adopted us from the slums of stupidity and gave us a home. Mother Yoga, Father Science you give us such protection and comfort in the Castle of your parental embrace, as we have never known.

In your Garden of nature's treasures, we meditate in awe, of the trees, the flowers and the waterfall. In the temple of appreciation, Using Mindful Movement with the breath, we dance and sing songs of Love and Appreciation to you, Mother Yoga and Father Science who adopted us.

Earl Dickey
April 21, 2019

CHAPTER 1

UPDATED YOGA NEEDED

Updating yoga isn't just an idea, thought to make yoga better by Upgrading. The concept of updating yoga is the result of a lifetime study of the human body's weaknesses, needs, strengths and studying negative results of some teachings.

Instructor / and creator of Shashi Yoga, Shashi Pottahil is a leading pioneer in the yoga field, with 45 years of experience. His teaching of Classical and Hatha yoga is a unique combination of science, health and spirituality.

Shashi has studied the impact of tools of learning, living, work, play, dress, social habits, eating, movement and lack of movement. All great projects are begun with a feasibility study. The impact of a project must be studied before or prior to the start of a project.

Shashi yoga was established only, after a lifetime of studying the needs of the body, as well as the effects of movement and lack of movement and the possibilities of negative effects. During the feasibility study, Shashi determined **two** misconceptions of yoga that must be clarified in the public's eyes.

1) **The thought that yoga is a strictly religious practice of eastern religions.**

    Shashi, assures us that yoga is available to people of any religion.

1

2)   **The idea that we need to be able to tie ourselves in a knot.**

Shashi, proves this wrong, by showing improved health for everyday people.

Shashi Yoga

Shashi is extremely proud of **three** important abilities he brings to updated yoga, he calls "Shashi Yoga:"

1)   **Firsthand knowledge of Sanskrit, that he can translate.**
2)   **The ability to simplify the language of science.**
3)   **Vast management experience to design a balanced east/west approach to yoga.**

In the fifteen years that I have known Shashi, he has always said that there are two types of body movement.

1)   **To use the body.**
2)   **To fix the body.**

Research data is mounting on the benefits of yoga, as confirmed by modern science all over the world. I agree that updated yoga is needed and updated yoga by Shashi Pottathil, as he teaches in his Shashi Yoga, is just what the science of yoga needs.

Updating an ancient science requires knowledge far above average. In fact, to update yoga, not only would one need to be well-versed in both the written and the practice forms of yoga, but would also need knowledge of science as related to the human body as well.

In addition to his knowledge of the human body, Shashi shares, a wealth of knowledge of animal bodies he observed in the jungles of India growing up, as related to both humans and animals in the science of movement.

Updating yoga would also require a professionally structured program, for maximum benefits.

Amazingly enough, Shashi also has management experience also among his many skills.

Shashi Yoga is a managed program, we are always reminded, that *"We never know when our last day is,"* while making reference to our death, people have quit – walked out! Because, Shashi often refers to the unknown time of our death. It is also hard for some people to see humans need of movement as unchanged, since primitive man.

"Mindful movement with the breath" is another of Shashi's most repeated quotes, as he continues to remind us of our need to move every part of our bodies every day.

I haven't heard Shashi speak of the "Laws of Life" as a set of Fifteen (15), or even mention them by name. Yet, I respect Shashi's approach to addressing the body's needs, with exercises that address the "Laws of Life".

Humans are all bound by the "Laws of Life" weather knowingly or unknowingly. Shashi Yoga is the only yoga I've seen that attend to so many areas of the "Laws of Life", which in itself credits Shashi Yoga, as being head and shoulders above schools that do not address the needs of the "Laws of Life".

The Laws of Life

(The Factors involving The Laws of Life)

This section alone is worth the price of the book and more. I feel since the body doesn't come with an instruction manual, "The Laws of Life Is a fantastic reminder of our body's needs."

When all is well in life, how little regard we have for our body's. In youth we are at our worst in taking chances and abusing our bodies.

This practice of neglecting our bodies is hard to break and continues until we have an accident or become ill in most cases. Even if we do wake up and start taking care of our bodies, before a serious accident or serious illness, we need to be able to distinguish if we are using the body, or fixing the body.

Here is a little help on how to determine if we are "fixing" the body, or "using" the body.

Generally, Daily activity is "using" the body. Sports or sleeping more than eight (8) hours a day, or sleep deprivation is also generally, "using" the body. Even over eating, is "using the body. We know that over eating is hard on the heart and the whole body suffers.

Families pass an awful lot of stress on to the rest of their family members as well. Shashi knows the story of stress runs deep, that's why before we begin our daily yoga practice, just before we begin to quiet our minds for a few minutes, before we start balancing or exercising; Shashi says, that we should close our eyes and *step out of the story,* (the stress we have bottled up inside us).

There are so many ways that we "use" our bodies, but Shashi's methods of "fixing" the body, are many also. Which include moderate eating, very little competitive sports and regularly practiced scientifically designed exercises, with the breath.

When Shashi directs his students to do these scientifically designed exercises, with the breath. I can't help but think of the ancient Tibetans belief, that the breath is the unseen winds, inside the body that propel the sails of the body's healing modalities, be they Electrical, Mechanical, Chemical, or even Spiritual and that our thoughts either help or hinder these currents of air, which drive the sails of our healing modalities.

The Laws of Life

Which govern, The Humans Species

1) **The Law of Breath**
We must breath or die.
Every cell in the body needs air.

2) **The Law of Harm**
Like an unwritten commandment for our treatment of others.
We should not harm, abuse or neglect our body.

3) **The Law of Balance and Gravity**
Balance and Gravity play a major role in the functioning and well-being of the body, which includes the brain.

4) **The Law of Movement**
The body needs movement.
The mind needs movement.
Even the air and the planets need movement.

5) **The Law of Nourishment**
All bodies have a bodily nourishment need be it air, water, food or sunlight.

6) **The Law of Rest**
The body needs Rest, Light and Darkness

7) **The Law of Waste Removal**
The body must dispose of waste toxins and some bacteria. The more we help the body with good hygiene the better.

8) **The Law of Attention and Accountability**
We must be aware and pay attention to our body's health and safety needs. Body abuse or neglect is punishable with pain and suffering. Guaranteed!

9) **The Law of Attraction and Reproduction**
Besides sexual attraction and procreation we can be an example of kindness, good health and good deeds.

10) **The Law of Fight Flight or Give Up**
The body's designer, installed such a strong inner force or drive for survival, which shows the 'importance' of the body and it's need for survival and well-being, Severe penalties as pain, suffering and death for the body's neglect or abuse is further proof of the body's "importance".

11) **The Law of Orderliness**
A tidy, necessary arrangement of objects that allows for unhampered functionality.

12) **The Law of Appreciation**
Without appreciation, we can have no love, no respect and therefore can-not inspire others to respect us. Without appreciation of the body, good health is short lived.

13) **The Law of Truth**
Truth is a companion of Fact. Which is essential for wisdom and knowledge. A Lie is an assault, or killing of the Truth.

14) **The Law of Time**
The body is a gift; **time** is a gift.

As nature has seasons, the body has seasons and **time** has seasons.

15) **The Law of Mortality**
The body dies.

Hopefully, "The Laws of Life" will remind you of the body's **need** to *live and function well*, that there are scientifically designed movements, or exercises that can maintain, or sometimes even "Fix" areas of the body, in need of special attention that are available.

CHAPTER 2

UPDATED YOGA FACILITIES NEEDED

Shashi Pottahil has introduced an updated practice of yoga that he calls Shashi Yoga.

While updating yoga we must also update the type of facility in which the science is taught.

Shashi believes in the science of yoga. He believes that this science should not be limited or condensed to an unflattering level, nor to a level minimizing yoga's ability to help fix or maintain the body. Universities are well aware of the importance of the image and updating a facility can make.

With a large amount of Shashi's family involved in Education and Science, he sees the need of presenting yoga in a professional manner, more so than most people involved in yoga.

Shashi's teaching facility is constantly being updated and with this constant updating, Shashi refers to his style and teaching facility as a "School of Yoga." The main yoga room where Shashi teaches his *mindful movement* with the breath" is like a school lab. Footwear is always removed and the facility is swept more frequently to insure a *clean room* for teaching his breathing exercises. Two open doors and an open window ensure good air circulation in the room.

For days when the weather might be a bit uncomfortable, Shashi has a good quality air conditioning unit, where the filters are replaced regularly. a fine heating and air conditioning service is always available.

For private and prenatal classes, a smaller room is available and this smaller room is also used for meditation. Like any good school Shashi has a library with many books that he selected himself.

All of his school's rooms are painted colors selected by an expert interior designer, with a knowledge of colors for schools and the work place. The colors provide the students with a good learning atmosphere and his school radiates an aura of professionalism.

Pregnant women who practice Yoga, work with well-trained Certified (RN) Nurses

Children, both handicapped and normal children, enjoy their respective classes, always by highly qualified teachers.

Seniors who enjoy classes with other seniors, can attend a class for seniors, taught by one of Shashi's advanced students.

Despite the huge number of students, amazingly, like any good counselor, Shashi makes time for students needing inspiration, counseling, direction or a friendly smile. Over the faint sound of background music, something drifts through the air… it feels like school to me.

It is said that curriculums are the foundation of a good school, perhaps Shishi's students recognize the wisdom in Shashi's school of Shashi Yoga, as many of Shash's students are from India with vast experience in yoga. Also, many students that are experienced in yoga come from other states and countries to learn Shashi Yoga. I do believe that one day in the near future Shashi's teachers will be more recognized for their knowledge of yoga, than they presently are.

CHAPTER 3

HAPPINESS YOGA

The Science of a Happy, Healthy, Balanced Life.

Hi! My name is Earl, my nick name is "Happy", my father's nick name was "Happy" also. My mother's nick name was "Bertie" because she was always singing. My Dad's older brother my uncle Martin Hansen spent maybe 30 years with the circus as a clown (called the man of a "Thousand Faces"), a contortionist, acrobat, etc. I come from a *very* HAPPY family. **I want to help you to be happy too.**

Nobody will go to any length to learn to do YOGA, if it doesn't make them feel good. We must find a key to feeling good about ourselves and yoga.

Yoga, is like a big key ring with loads of keys for every thing imaginable.

- GOOD HEALTH
- FLEXIBILITY
- SELF CONTROL
- GOAL SETTING
- BALANCE
- MEMORY ENHANCEMENT
- SEEING HUMOR IN LIFE

How about "Happiness" now, in this life? As long as there is breath there is hope.

As we enter into and advance in a study such as yoga, we need to bring a "Happy Attitude", so when the body enjoys yoga, you too will enjoy your time doing yoga. Besides, a Happy attitude helps to give us mental strength to continue our exercises, even if we are just plain lazy. For years it has also been well known, that a happy attitude promotes good health, both physically and mentally.

There seems to be somewhat of a promise in writings on yoga, that the regular practice of Yoga will take us to the Higher Brain and it will even open the gates to wisdom.

As "X" is the missing number in mathematical equations and "Sugar" is the ingredient that brings a smile and helps the medicine go down. A "Happy Attitude" is a necessary ingredient for bland, or even sour tasting projects to be done or learned. Not that Yoga is a bland, or a sour tasting undertaking, but besides our moments of laziness or procrastination life and loved ones often will put an enormous pull on us, not seeing our Yoga time as important.

The Science of the "Yoga Smile"

(Gateway To Happiness)

The art of the "Yoga Smile" goes even deeper than one may realize. The Yoga Smile as written here, is my blend of segments of ancient and modern exercises, positive thinking, meditations and scientific knowledge.

Let's start the study of the practice, of the "Yoga Smile", scientifically, as a learned pattern of living, we perform these exercises in front of a mirror, as a way to get to know ourselves better.

In a study called Lally's Study (on Google), it is said that not all habits are formed in a certain time frame. "That it took from 18 days to 254 days to form a new habit".

Training the mind and body for Happiness should be started as a meditation, then expanded into our everyday activities in life.

This exercise is an *open eye meditation*, that you will be able to do later in your garden, or going for a walk in your everyday life. It is as simple as feeling the sun or rain on your face, or a gentle breeze that sends a pleasant tickle down the spine and throughout the body, to the very tips of our nerve endings in our fingers and toes.

The Start:

We begin by standing in front of the bathroom mirror. **Eyes always open.** Older or sickly students, may chose to hold the edge of the sink, or the stand that holds the sink. Since we plan to visit with the image in the mirror a while. Preferably, just after bathing and grooming.

> Smile! Smile Moore! Laugh!
> (note how good it feels.)
> Let your mind explore this feeling in depth.
>
> Sincerely, compliment yourself like…
> "Gosh! Your looking great!"
> Smile More Now And Say,
> "Thanks! *I Feel Great Too*"

Now, <u>feel</u> your smile, like a great waterfall of happiness coursing through your entire body.

Next search for Sincerity in the eyes. You Must learn to *fill the eyes*, with Sincere Happiness that you can feel in your face as you smile. Practice expanding and feeling that

Sincere Happiness, spreading from the eyes throughout your entire face and body.

Never, Never under estimate the importance of the mouth's need for sincerity in the smile, if we are to obtain true happiness.

As we searched for sincerity in the Eyes, now we search for sincerity in the Mouth. As you look into the mirror at your mouth, would you believe a sales person with a mouth like that? We must determine how to direct the mouth for our best smile.

As the mouth provides us with a place to take in, our life sustaining food and water. The Mouth also provides us with two positions that we can choose. We can choose to wear a smile and feel good, or we can wear a frown and feel bad. How we breath, hold ourselves, or move our bodies, eyes and mouth are no less important.

As we consciously chose in our mirror exercise, _how to Look_ Happy, for we must _look happy_ and _feel happy_ TO BE HAPPY and to be able to direct the power of the smile from our eyes, throughout the body. Next we direct the Sincere Smile of the Mouth, to do like the eyes, we expand the smile from the mouth and direct it to flow in a powerful torrent throughout the body.

I'm sure you will think...Wow! This does feel Great!

However, my friend this is just the start.

Now:

- Practice a Chuckle (a gentle laugh).
- Practice Beaming (smiling with the eyes only).

Smiling

Watch the Breath flow in through both nostrils and out through the mouth, maybe four times.

Take a deep Breath through both nostrils and exhale evenly through the mouth.

Take another Breath through both nostrils and exhale evenly through the mouth.

Still smiling, breath normal and watch the breath, Eyes Always Open. Continue to feel Happy while observing your breathing pattern and notice the spread of happiness throughout your body.

Shake the belly as if chuckling, we are now shifting our attention from the breath, to the Smile Beams radiating throughout the body. Shake the belly again, notice the power and choppiness of the smile beam and how you are in control. Feel and know that you are happy. Say I am Happy! I Feel Happy! I Look Happy! I am Happy! There is always the need to Give Thanks for happiness. Say, I Give Thanks! I Give Thanks! I Give Thanks!

CHAPTER 4

THE EGG

Personally, the Egg to me is the best symbol of updated yoga, more so than a person in meditation. The Egg to me represents the womb of life even the ancients held the Egg in high esteem, being the most sculptured subject and the oldest sculptures on the earth, often with unknown carvings and writings with no translation, even today.

The Egg where life begins. Shashi often begins his class lecture by anatomizing the unity of all the body, limbs, trunk and internal organs, also often describing the body's marvelous scientific beginning from a single egg…fertilized, then traced by science, through its various steps of development in the womb.

Science is always documenting its observations. Science documents cells continuous division, proving the body's limbs are not separate from the trunk of the body, no more than the limbs of a tree are separate additions to the trunk of the tree.

It would be quite foolish indeed to have separate doctors for the trunk of the tree, a specialist for the limbs of the tree and a specialist for the young leaves and a specialist for the older leaves.

To me it stands to reason, that IF the entire body, mind, bones, muscles, nerves and organs NEEDED to be considered separately, for medical treatment, we would have been born with separate umbilical cords instead of a single umbilical cord.

The body is so inter-connected, neither medicine nor yoga should neglect the fact that the body is a single unit and not all health problems are born where they first appear.

Shashi uses the example of life in the womb as a separate life, as at one stage, we are a fish in the water of the womb. When we exit the womb, we take on a human form and we cease to breath water and begin to breath air.

Shashi likens birth, to dying from our watery life in the womb and being reborn in the air, as a human with no knowledge of our life in the womb; not knowing if we are a snake or a buffalo. Which is an interesting concept that I have heard before. I have also seen the comparison to a caterpillar being reborn as a butterfly.

Egg Candling

My mother grew up on a farm, and for a while when I was a kid my parents had a small farm. As a kid I recall a little farm life. My parents had irrigation ditches for watering. They had irrigation ditches that provided water for the different rows of corn, beans, peas, lettuce, etc. until all the vegetables were watered.

When my parents had their little farm, we had some chickens too. My parents took a cardboard box and made a small hole on one side, Maybe an inch or so in diameter. They had an electric light inside the box.

The room was darkened and my parents would hold eggs up to the hole, in a process called candling (perhaps the term was used from a time when candles were used for this process).

Egg candling determines the condition of air cell, yoke and white of the egg. Candling also detects bloody whites, blood spots and also enables observation of germ development.

I see Shashi Yoga as a light to view the condition of the student's health, in the Egg or womb of life, as well as the health needs of the student.

In his yoga class, Shashi talks of the of the body and the fluids, being supplied to the body's areas in need and the amount of fluids needed. When it comes to the body's needs, the body is far smarter than we give the body credit for.

Shashi always praises the wisdom of the body and tells us to learn to listen to the body. There are times though when the body is lazy, or wants to procrastinate, or times of being tired, or that we are illogical, these are often indications of oxygen deprivation, electrical, magnetic, or fluid imbalance. All of which yoga can help. But if they continue, see your doctor.

Shashi Yoga provides excellent direction for the body's health, his managed movement with the breath has brought him students from all over the world.

Scrambled, poached, over easy, over hard; as we might select our breakfast wants each morning, Sharshi determines the classes' yoga *needs"* for the day. Tomorrow, Shashi may feel that we have other body needs to fix, that we may have other issues to address. Because there is so much to fix or maintain, we can't do all of our scientific movements every day, because of time.

Shashi is always telling his class that the body has millions of ways to move and that the body must not be limited to only a few basic movements, **or the Body will Lose Thousands of ways to move …and faster still every year or two as we grow older and become less active.**

Speeds are a necessary part of Shashi's teachings. Sometimes, usually the start of our daily exercises, we begin slow, slow, and with caution, so sensitive areas like the neck, spine, knees and sore or, tender areas are not hurt.

As the body is warmed up speeds of movement can be increased, except the neck or injured areas, which should never reach speeds three or four.

The Magic figure 8

Like the Egg, areas of the body are sometimes sore or fragile, needing to be treated like a thin shelled egg, or flower (Shashi often refers to the body as a flower or a soap bubble). Besides building flexibility and balance, yoga helps strengthen this egg shell, flower, or bubble, known as the body.

In addition to exercise movements and circles as rotating one's head, body or limbs, there is a scientifically designed movement, or exercise used in Shashi Yoga besides circles and rotations of the head, arms, body or legs. That is drawing the figure Eight (8) with the body or body part. Which can be done in many directions laying down or standing up, but Shashi Yoga does it very slow.

It is not unusual to have one side of the body stronger than the other, it is the student's eventual aim, to make both sides of the body equal in strength and movement. If we are mindful and faithful in our yoga practice, we will experience our body's health blossoming, like the flower that it is.

From the womb or egg of the Higher brain our greatest thoughts are born. Faithful yoga practice, will one day hatch an experience of good health, peace and joy never thought possible.

CHAPTER 5

THE BREATH

Legends abound about breath. Without direction the Breath can be likened to an uneducated child lacking discipline.

With direction, a child can become a scientist, a doctor, or a lawyer. With an education, a child can take a mind originally likened to that of a maddened monkey and direct and guide the mind into areas of science and technology, never before explored or traveled.

So too, as we learn Shashi Yoga, we educate the body and the breath. Because of some Yogi's Educated Breath. Yogi's have been known to have fantastic health, fantastic minds and super-human abilities.

Access to the Higher Brain is said to be known by yogis of India, and Shashi Yoga is said to be capable of taking us to the Higher Brain. Shashi has yogi's in his family who have passed much of this knowledge on to Shashi.

The Science of Breath

Breathing techniques are some of the ways of educating the breath and strengthening the lungs. You will find that there are formulas and laws in the science of breath.

Shashi likes to relate many interesting facts about breath. For Example:

- **Butterflies live but 28 days perhaps, counting their life's breaths in seconds**
- **Rain Flies live six hours perhaps counting their life's breaths in micro-seconds.**
- **Dogs live maybe 8 to 10 years breathing very fast, maybe 60 breaths a minute.**
- **Turtles live maybe 200 years, but breathing only once in four (4) minutes. This seems to confirm that slower calmer breathing patterns are rewarded with longer lives.**

As scientists in biology use dissection and cutting apart of specimens, to explain their point in biology, Shashi breaks down the breath and the breaths scientific structure and the roll of the body, as described in India's ancient Sanskrit texts.

Shashi teaches many techniques of breathing untaught by other yoga schools, one example, is Breathing Speeds: Breathing fast in cold weather to warm the body and breathing slow to cool the body in warm weather.

Shashi teaches many, standing, sitting and moving, breathing exercises; he also teaches breathing techniques with one nostril, both nostrils, breathing with alternate nostrils and techniques of when and what breathing exercises to do, with the mouth.

One interesting technique used in Shashi Yoga is folding the tongue and drinking air, as though through a straw. **We learn here also, the importance of raising the arms above the heart, during some breathing exercises, as it aids us in breathing with different lobes of the lungs.**

For maximum benefit of the breath. Shashi Yoga teaches ... The "Need" to clean the tubes and "How".

Shashi Yoga teaches the cleaning of our breathing tubes of bacteria and toxins, with air and sound for maximum benefits of the air we breathe, addressing areas where no chemicals can reach and few yoga schools go.

Cleaning our tubes is another step in educating ourselves to the need and the fact, that there are methods to maintain a healthier body and to reduce germs, toxins and bacteria from our bodies.

I personally am very impressed and like the idea that Shashi Yoga teaches, the digestion of the air we breathe and bringing this digested air down to the cellular level of the body.

People outside of yoga have no idea how much there is to learn about the science of breath. Sleeping, working, playing, meditating, bathing, eating, even stress and our attitude all effect our breath.

Shashi Yoga explains, how we unconsciously hold our breath when we are angry, depriving our bodies of much needed oxygen, also when we engage in negative thinking, we unconsciously hold our breath causing us to operate our bodies at an unhealthy frequency.

Yogis realize how our bodies vibrate to different frequencies. As we engage in different activities or inactivity, the condition of our health can be changed dramatically. In fact, Yogis say that our health can be improved when we learn to control our breath and direct oxygen to the areas of the body desperately in need of healing.

The healing ability of oxygen is becoming more and more recognized in science and medicine. For example, people with decompression sickness, or the bends, (from coming up to fast from diving deep in the ocean), are treated with special measured amounts of oxygen, to stabilize them. Under some health conditions, science has found great results in using oxygen therapy for healing.

Modern Science, is still learning about oxygen's effects on both the outer and inner area of the body, in their labs and from ancient texts.

Fortunately, people like Shashi's ancestors handed down information on yoga and the breath, as well as teaching how to read and use these ancient texts.

Cleaning the Body

The importance of cleaning the body can never be over-emphasized. Brushing the teeth, is about the extent of our attention to daily cleaning an interior portion of the body. We give no thought to cleaning our throats, or nasal cavities.

Germs, toxins and bacteria not only exists in our mouths. Our germs, bacteria and toxins also exist (often thriving) in our throats, nasal passages and sinus cavities. Mouth washes should not be used, as mouth washes are harmful to friendly bacteria.

Our throats, nasal passages, and sinus cavities need a daily flushing with a little salty water and some breathing techniques.

In India a metal devise is used to scrape the tongue gently. This simple yet important organ is often ignored here in the west. Though some of us here in the west would do some tongue exercises and then scrape our tongues gently with a simple spoon.

Fixing the body

The body and the mind's happiest time together is fixing the body and fixing the brain.

We find there are two types of body movement.

1)   To use the body.
2)   To fix the body.

As harmony and some quality time are needed for a good family life, the body needs some quality time with the mind too. Shashi assures us that mindful movement with the breath can and will take us to fantastic heights of good health and then into the Higher Brain, with its' vast wisdom and joy.

In youth or good health, we have a tendency to only use the body, as the body in youth is usually free of pain or detects no discomfort. Like money, good health is usually wasted without the twin spotlights of knowledge and attention.

To neglect our health, our body then is destined to have pain and suffering and we are just waiting for a crisis.

Fixing or maintaining the body is not quick and is not easy, while sometimes it's just too late, for fixing the body. Yoga and modern medicine can only do so much, to fix or repair damaged bodies.

As we bring this chapter on the Breath to a close; We need to remember, **Shashi says, "when we have a question about the body,**

Ask a good scientist, or better yet make science your hobby."

CHAPTER 6

THE BODY

(Designed and Built with Love)

How many ways can our body's creator say, "I Love You!"?

How many times does the body's creator need to tell us, that not only is our souls precious to Him / Her, but our *bodies* are precious to our creator as well?

If every cell in these Amazing Bodies of ours, has a fraction of the survival instincts that we are consciously aware of as, Fight or Flight with warning systems involving our senses such as Sight, Touch, Sound, Reproduction, etc. within the total physical body.

Imagine, Science tells us that every cell in the body, has all the needs and functions of an entire human body, including the survival instinct. **if each cell has all these survival instincts and we multiply that number by all the cells in our bodies, that is a lot of ways our creator says physically He / She loves our bodies, *as well as our souls* and wants us to us to survive... and to maintain our bodies.**

With any fraction of logic, we must conclude that the body has a far greater value to our Creator than Ancient or Modern Texts relate to us... As Shashi so aptly put's it "Maintaining our bodies is not an option".

Continuing the subject of our responsibility and honor to care for, what must be the greatest manifestation of Divine Love for us imaginable. Yes, that's when the Creator created US.

Every molecule, every atom, in our bodies are vibrating, dancing and we have the honor to choreograph their movement to a healthy frequency, with Yoga. Allowing us to shape our bodies and design our bodies movements for the stage of life.

Religion says, that our Creator dwells within the hearts of each and every one of us. If so, all the more reason to respect our bodies Now, and to do yoga. Let's Imagine an imaginary window in our heart and as we peer inside the window, we see our creator at a huge drafting table designing ways to say that He / She Loves us and where to put the world' s greatest doctor and Where to place the world's greatest pharmacy.

Perhaps we would see a smile, as our Creator decides where in our bodies and where in our brains to place the world's greatest computers. We could almost hear an audible Uh-ha (yet sad) as our Creator determines a place for a *Courtroom of Bodily Affairs*, With the world's greatest Judge to hear every complaint of neglect and abuse, of the body.

I believe simplicity in a story book fashion, is not only a great way for children to grasp an idea. Adults also can enjoy a simplified visual form of presenting an idea. Personally, I really enjoy the Tibetan's concept of the Breath's function in healing in the body. **Tibetans say that, "the breath is the unseen winds inside the body, that propel the sails of the body's healing modalities, be they electrical, mechanical, chemical or even spiritual and our thoughts either help or hinder these currents of air, which drive the sails, of our healing modalities."**

As we return to the subject of neglect and abuse. We have no right to neglect a child or even a pet in our care. We must admit that our bodies are like a most loyal child, servant or in some cases a slave that we have no right to abuse or neglect. Weather the Creator has designed our bodies for us, or for some divine plan on the stage of life. We have no right to neglect our bodies that we enjoy.

I believe that our Creator has installed a Judge in the *Court of Bodily Affairs,* loyal to the Creator, a Judge that can't be bribed.

No Doctor, no crooked Lawyer, can reverse a ruling where bodily abuse has been determined. Pain and suffering is the currency to pay fines, in the *Court of Bodily Affairs.*

Shashi loves to maintain and even hone the bodies memory skills and give credit to the bodies many facets, that work so well together. Even giving credit to cells with a three (3) day life span, yet they pass on all they know before they die.

Shashi not only talks about, but trains the body's amazing memory and ability, to react to dangers in a flash. Such as a truck pulling out in front of us. We immediately put on the brake. Or if a child or pet runs out in front of us, we immediately hit the brake.

I like to think of the cells in the body, with super quick reaction time for a single purpose; as being even more than Body Intellect (but a form of "Swarm Intelligence"). I have always been fascinated to see flocks of birds, or hundreds of bees in flight turn left, turn right, go high, go low and even reverse direction as though a single body. Years later I see it referred to as "Swarm Intelligence".

I hope that this chapter or this book, kindles a flame of Yoga passion in you that you practice enough Yoga, that you enjoy a long, happy, healthy, pain free, life.

CHAPTER 7

YOGA SAFETY

Some people have gone against their Doctor's advice and have had great results. Although both Shashi and I are different people, neither Shashi nor I would ever suggest doing anything against the advice of a doctor of medicine. Everything in this book is written as a *preventive therapy,* to help us maintain a healthy body, or to help us improve our health.

This updated yoga does not claim to be a *cure-all,* in competition with modern medicine. For over 40 years, Shashi has done his best to work with modern medicine and to present the blessings of knowledge gained from both, Modern Science and the Ancient Science of Yoga as well.

Shashi has gone to great lengths to provide a wide range of "Baby Steps" in degrees, speeds, and the amount of repetitions in both body movements and breathing techniques.

The Ego

When Shashi has a health issue involving himself or a member of his family, he informs his students that he is going to seek medical counsel, regarding that particular health issue. For example, a while back he tripped on a chair and the soreness lingered. He informed his students of the issue and that he was going to have it checked out. Shashi recommended to his students, that any time a student hurts themselves, they should not hesitate to have it checked out by a doctor.

Shashi points out that some people have such egos that they don't go to a doctor when they need to. Telling his students that letting their egos keep them from going to the doctor is foolish.

The ego is often the weakest link in an otherwise strong safety program. The ego can shut-off the hearing so that we don't hear safety instructions. The ego can also blind us to dangers we don't want to see…Perhaps like the man who built his house on sand.

Attempting shortcuts and laziness, are also dangers to maintaining safety. Cheating the body of proper conditioning by attempting shortcuts, or being lazy is not smart, nor is it safe. Major athletes do warm-up exercises we should do warm-up exercises too.

A wide range of "Baby Steps" has been created by Shashi for Yoga Safety. Yoga by degrees, speeds and amounts of repetitions in both body movement and breathing techniques, are excellent ways to manage your Yoga routine safely.

Yoga students should be sure to inform the instructor of any health issues before starting a program like yoga, even though yoga programs are less taxing than a lot of programs, all yoga schools aren't the same.

We should never exceed our comfort range of motion and never allow someone to force us beyond our range of motion. Forcing someone beyond their natural range of motion has been the cause of countless injuries around the world.

We should do sets of exercises, rather than a large number of any exercises. Instead of doing 10 or 20 repetitions, we might do two sets of five first, for a goal of 10 repetitions. For a goal of 20 repetitions, we might do four sets of five repetitions.

Suggestion:

If exercises are kept at even number counts, there is the advantage that if the student is sick, or if a new student can't

do 20 (twenty) repetitions, they can do only 10 repetitions. If they are really sick or weak rather than disrupting a good routine and stop yoga, or postpone starting yoga, they might do only 5 (Five) repetitions. Always try to establish and maintain good habits for your practice.

When we are holding Yoga Positions, it is best to hold the position for a specific time. One may count to one self, like one thousand one (1,001), one thousand two (1,002), one thousand three (1,003), one thousand four (1,004), one thousand five (1,005). If the position was only done on one side, we should turn to the opposite side and repeat the hold count for that side.

Eating less than an hour before doing Yoga is not safe. Not to eat before any strenuous activities, is always recommended by doctors, perhaps for more reasons than we know.

Partner Yoga is not recommended for many reasons, such as one partner is usually in better condition and harmonizing with a partner can be a distraction, from concentrating on your own body's safety.

If the wrist won't bend to a 45-degree angle, then don't put weight on it such as hand stands or push-ups, as you could suffer a serious injury.

When lowering the head below the waist, had your eye doctor told you not to do it, then don't do it. You could be putting your eyes in severe danger, bringing a strong blood and body fluid pressure to the head.

Head, neck and spine rotations, should always be started slowly, because of the presence of delicate nerves that any quick, or sudden movements can cause severe even permeant damage, or even body paralysis.

Wall Yoga is not recommended on a regular basis, as it puts quite a strain on the joints and is most often used as a test, for finding areas of the body an instructor may choose to focus on, for a student's yoga needs.

Slipperiness, is a situation we must be mindful of. Socks, or blankets on wood floors are extremely slippery and vary dangerous, when you detect a dangerous situation, never take a chance.

Videos or books to learn yoga without an instructor, is not a wise way to save money, ask your doctor if they think it is safe for you.

The best way that I can think of to close this chapter on "Safety", is a variation of one of Shashi's most famous quotes. **"When you have a question on science ask a good scientist. Or better yet make science your hobby."**

Safety is so important in life, both to ourselves and to our families, I think "Safety" should be an important Hobby of ours, at work and at Play.

Have fun with Yoga and stay safe!

CHAPTER 8

GROUNDING

(Being in the Present)
(Observing Earth's Life Force)

Grounding, in Shashi's teachings is usually *the science of being in the present.* Grounding provides so much, as grounding implies a connection with the **ground/ earth**, in fact the **planet.** Vast benefits await us when we learn to tap the earth's **Life Force.**

Being Grounded implies that one is **focused on the present, an object, subject, matter or even an action** and that **Possible distractions have been removed, from the window of our minds, or how we are viewing the matter being focused upon.**

Other terms for being *in the present or being focused* are, **Being Anchored, or Being in the "Now!", Being Centered, or Being in the Present, or Paying Attention.**

Not being Grounded would be. **Like Daydreaming while Driving, letting your mind wander** during a **lecture or conversation,** or allowing **distractions as by sight, sound etc. to interrupt actions or thoughts. In fact, Not paying complete attention.**

Libraries are full of books with lists of benefits when connecting with the earth, where we reap the benefits of magnetic fields, wonderful energies and gravity. Vast benefits await us when we are grounded in the present, say numerous teachers. Benefits galore, await us when we make Gravity our Tutor for better balance.

So often people say that we should strive to be in the present, but use the term so loosely and often like an incomplete sentence... Unlike Shashi who explains inner and outer benefits, of being grounded in the present.

Yoga is a science that for centuries, has dealt with our need to be grounded and to be in the present. We need to know the depth and security of our roots of learning, that our roots of learning are secured to the stones of facts and faith, together with stretching our arms of mindfulness which would enable us to reach the Higher Brain.

Amazingly, our minds cannot only leap continents and dimensions at a single bound. Our energies and our brains can leap worlds and galaxies at a single bound.

Shashi says that a reporter once asked him what he wanted most.

Shashi said that he told the reporter that "He wanted most to make his students enlightened".

If the human mind can direct it's thought patterns to sub-atomic depths, sub-atomic dimensions, as well as expand our thought patterns to outer dimensions, outer worlds, outer galaxies...as though our world is but an atom. Then what great amounts of good could humans accomplish, if humans could control and harness their fantastic abilities?

Other than Yoga, I see no means of grounding our minds from the hurricane winds of distraction, causing wandering minds and restless bodies.

Martial artists often appear to have good grounding, but they need to constantly consider different confrontation possibilities. The intense nature of confrontation causes them to lose some of their grounding abilities.

Grounding as in Yoga training, has benefits that reach far and wide, as being able to enhance our skills and senses, such as Balance and the ability to Focus.

When I was a teenager, I had friends who made antennas for the government and complex underground sonar and complex electronic equipment, some were heavily into metaphysics and spoke of how Science, Yoga and Metaphysics when tied together, great scientific achievements of unimaginable heights, would be at mankind's fingertips.

Nikola Tesla, brilliant Serbian-American engineer and physicist born in 1856 and died in 1943. Nikola Tesla claimed, "that the ground or earth contained enough electrical power, to provide free energy to the entire world." I consider Nikola Tesla, the greatest mind ever. If Mr. Tesla said that there is that much power in the ground, claims of benefits of grounding must be every bit as important as other Scientists claim.

Grounding is a form of accessing earth's energies with yoga, or metaphysics and helps hold the mind in the "Now" and is said to be an ancient study. Shashi Yoga makes no claim, to the miracle abilities of the ancients, but it is great to see Shashi having such a wide range of success.

Great benefits of earths' properties await us through the science of grounding, the ground supplies us with minerals for our body's needs, powerful minerals and substances, used in science and medicine. The Life force's power emanating from Vegetation, Foods grown both on and in the earth, and the vibratory benefits of Jewels, Minerals, and Metals like Gold and Silver should be no surprise.

There is great value in taping the power of the earth, through the power of grounding. Grounding, may be accessing the power of light, sound, electronics, magnetics, vegetation, thermo or ..., the benefits of grounding are many and along with meditation and yoga open doors of many possibilities. The frequency of the earth, and the frequencies of life, can be used to reach the Higher Brain and the "Castle of Human Potential".

Some Yoga practitioners consider their bodies as being an electrical power supply and send a wire or metal stake, or their feet, into the ground or earth (With their minds) to complete an electrical circuit, they believe this circuit will better enable their bodies and their minds to tap earth's unseen energies, for better balance and to create a spiritual or metaphysical tool.

These Yoga Practitioners say our imaginary roots are like screws or springs twisting turning deeper and deeper, they even encircle rocks and cement. As water energizes roots they thicken and expand, crushing would-be deterrents, while stretching also upward in slow motion and growth.

Perhaps visualizing ourselves with roots works well, because scientists and old yoga texts are right, that our DNA does contain elements and memory of vegetation in our DNA makeup.

Not only do animals provide us with lessons for maintaining our health and well-being, trees and vegetation have lessons for us also, both above and below ground, that yoga has long documented and taught.

Visualizing trees and plants and their fantastic root system, is an excellent technique for grounding one self.

Be Present While Driving

Grounding is not only needed for good balance, grounding also aids us in keeping the mind from wandering, so we can be in the present.

Being in the present is important, especially when driving. True, the mind loves to engage in visualization, or multiple thoughts at the same time. However, there are so many things happening at one time while driving, that it is best to make every effort to be alert to every facet of our driving, including the ever-changing traffic and ever-changing surroundings, weather conditions and road hazards as well.

Like on our computers, as we drive there are so many situations, like pop-ups, that appear suddenly and demand our attention.

Granted… We live busy and stressful lives…but for our own safety and the safety of others, we need to remain mindful of our driving. **For Heavens' Sake…don't do visualization exercises while driving.**

Living in The Now

The beauty of grounding is, that grounding is truly the art of being in the present. Only by accepting the fact that we are living in the now and must focus upon and deal with, all that occurs involving us in the present

Our imaginary roots may not be as imaginary as we think (Just because we can't see these roots doesn't mean that some kind of unseen link to the ground does not exist.) If an umbilical cord can exist between a mother and a child, why can't a type of unseen umbilical cord exist, between the earth and each of us humans, as a bond might exist between a mother and child? A person that losses a limb and experiences feeling where the limb would be, a phantom (unseen) limb is said to exist. (Is it really just the nerves that once lead to the limb that was removed? And how about once conjoined twins having telepathic unity? Or a mother and child's telepathic unity?)

Shashi Yoga, seldom speculates and leans most heavily on yoga as Shashi knows it and the accepted findings of modern science. Until you explore Shashi Yoga on your own, you are missing the Shashi Yoga view. Interestingly, Shashi's Teachers even view Yoga a little different from Shashi. When the opportunity arrives, do take some classes from Shashi Personally.

When I was writing this book, the computer ate a number of my chapters several times. Anxious to finish, and being computer stupid I sent off hand written versions often incomplete, hoping that professionals would be able to finish my book for me (It just didn't work out.). Without recordings of Shashi's actual teachings, which at this time <u>is not permitted</u>, nor did Shashi have the time for long interviews. Hopefully these writings show that even from my view, the reader will see the value of Shashi yoga and his drive to update yoga.

We can't help but marvel at the fantastic composition of the human being. Spirit, Mind, Body and Wow! (Wow! Might be a good word for Human Potential.)

As we read this book on Updating Yoga, we can't help but praise the bodies' fantastic abilities to maintain and heal it-self. Like the saying that we have within our bodies the world's greatest Doctor and the world's Greatest Pharmacy (etc.).

Now that we have arrived at Chapter 8, our chapter on Grounding. **We might begin to see the immense *potential of the human body being* expanded by accessing earth's energies, doing Yoga and accessing our own Higher Brain.**

For years earth has been called *the third rock from the sun.* But, Oh! What a rock it is!!!

- Mysterious elements, with many unknowns.
- Mysterious energies, also with many unknowns.
- Mysterious qualities, that boggle the minds of science.

Earth is our mother, the rarest of planets in countless galaxies. One of the very few earths (rocks in the heavens able to support life as we know it.)

Science, scans the heavens daily searching, searching, with their most powerful telescopes, for signs of a planet, like the Cosmic Jewel that we call Earth. With all of Science's High Technology, as we, the public understand. Science makes no mention of another Cosmic Jewel like the planet Earth.

Both Yoga and Earth have oceans of powers to be accessed for improving our lives and the planet's needs. Like the song "Rain Drops keep falling on my head". Science is always finding more and more *"blessings of Knowledge"* gifts from mother earth.

CHAPTER 9

HARMONIZING

In Chapter 8 our last chapter we discussed "Grounding". In this chapter we will discuss "Harmony in Health", as Yoga is truly a master at blending, mixing and balancing the various segments of the body, like a music conductor can blend, mix and balance the music from various instruments in a symphony. Yoga can Harmonize the health of all the body's limbs and organs to operate at the necessary frequencies required for good health.

Blending and mixing has become quite the Science and Technology, where sound technicians, use mixing boards for blending and mixing the music at musical events.

In health a far more serious approach to the blending, mixing and harmonizing all the elements involved in a healthy human body. Yes, that serious approach, is the science of yoga.

We find in sound or light, any time that there is more than one sound or more than one colored light at the same time, if their frequencies aren't in harmony, it can be very annoying to the point of even making one sick.

Yoga recognizes the necessity of **balancing our thought patterns,** yoga also recognizes *the dangers of not harmonizing* **negative thought frequencies**, to counter their negativity. Shashi Yoga is always telling us to step away from these thought patterns. **As Shashi says, "Step out of the story!"**

Light, sound and thought patterns, in fact all of our senses, even our sense of smell, all have frequencies that

need to be in harmony for good health. Yoga can help balance these frequencies to a Harmonic level. Internal Organs are extremely sensitive to these frequencies. Seeing Shashi Yoga address the need of Yoga, for the internal organs, is great to see.

It's said that everything is vibrating at some frequency be it trees, buildings, furniture, metals. All are vibrating at an atomic or sub atomic frequency. History tells us that the sounding of a trumpet brought down the walls of Jericho. Science tells us and even demonstrates, how sound can shatter glass. Science even tells us the frequency that shatters glass.

When I was in school, I was told the benefits of different colored vegetables and again, when I was last in the hospital, I was told the need of a balanced plate. All this reminds me color is frequency, color is Life.

When yoga brings the body into a state of good health, Yoga is not only balancing frequencies, yoga is harmonizing these frequencies with a science sometimes referred to as Harmonics.

In this book I am doing my best not to give it any religious leaning, although, the Ancients believed that Yoga not only balanced the body and the mind, but also brought a balance to the spirit, believing yoga brought a balance between, The Body, Mind and Spirit (sometimes referred to as Body, Mind and Soul).

Never in the history of yoga, has such an opportunity existed as at this time, where science can validate or prove the effectiveness of the science of yoga.

Frequencies to Harmonize With

Harmonizing with the wrong roll model, just to fit into a popular social group, even for a few years is not a smart thing to do. Habits are hard to break and bad habits that affect the health can't always be corrected and if they are, it might take years of yoga and seeing a medical doctor to regain even some of one's lost health.

The world has changed and Harmonizing with a social group who is health conscious, or finding a health minded mentor, is easier than ever to find.

Groups of health conscious or likeminded people, are everywhere you turn, even without checking the internet. Good health practices are more socially acceptable, with even the news media promoting good health practices more than ever.

Good health practitioners are emitting such a strong frequency of proof and truthfulness at yoga's effectiveness, one might say Yoga's Aura of healthfulness has reached new heights in popularity. People are experiencing wonderful results to their practice of yoga. People are witnessing great things in yoga. Even the media has shown the spotlights of their attention on yoga and the good that Yoga has done and is doing far and wide.

It's been almost twenty years now, after Shashi quit his job to pursue his dream and start teaching his style of yoga full time.

Sometimes life's situations and our goals require a great deal of creativity. As the strings on a fine stringed instrument are tightened and loosened for tuning. Shashi has fine-tuned the segments of yoga for each part of the body to create a harmonic flow of energy, realizing movement creates energy and energy creates movement.

Success whether in school, the work place, even successful spiritual, or family lives require effort and sacrifices. We must often deal with difficult people and difficult situations. We learn to make concessions and we learn the art of cooperation.

Now, if we want good to excellent health, we have to engage in some selfishness, self-discipline and still harmonize with our families—whew! But you can do it.

Shashi says, that he has had people start yoga, leave, and come back, many years later. Some people never make it back.

One person wanted to spend at least two days before they died with Shashi. But their doctor wouldn't let them.

The cell and the cells' digestion, is almost a constant part of Shashi's lectures on the depth of yoga. Also, Shashi often states that *mindful movement with the breath* is a major key to Shashi Yoga and that a healthy body in **harmony** with it-self and the universe, **can only then access the frequency of the higher brain.**

CHAPTER 10

BALANCE

Balance must be one of our parent's greatest gifts after the gift of life. In most cases our parents spent a lot of time and effort teaching us to walk. Next, they taught us to balance safety versus danger, our parents taught us Language, so we might have balance between home and the community and to learn the rules of home and the rules of the community.

Human children are said to remain in the proverbial nest longer than any other animal on the earth. Why?

When humans first decided to walk upright, it was then decided the need to educate their young in the art of "Balance". Before teaching their young hunting and gathering, balance was needed to stand upright as tall as possible to detect danger. They would teach their young how to balance on two legs while observing how safe or dangerous the area was, as they moved about could have been the child's second lesson, in the art of balance.

Maneuverability may very well have been the child's next lesson in balance, as the child learns to climb trees, to climb cliffs and maneuver themselves upon slippery rocks.

Even in modern life, there is still no food, no pill, no shot for balance. Only for ear infections or ear wax can doctors help, when balance is disrupted.

In the wild, we would be dead shortly after a balance problem, because without balance we become so helpless. Only having two legs to walk upon requires more balance than we remember. We forget the time and effort it takes for a child to learn to walk. Only people who practice balance as entertainers can realize the work involved in maintaining our balance, especially as we age.

Balance has always been important for our survival in history, as well as balance in the wild, such as in the jungle. Life or death always hinged on balance. Shashi says, "Even animals with a limp become other animal's prey in the jungle". Little or no balance, or even slowness, would not allow one to get food, or chase even slow, moving prey. Death would be near and certain with not being able to get food or run from the enemy.

Yoga to the rescue

Balance—one word, so many uses. Even in yoga, we have a lot of ways that the word balance applies to the body. Balance is a foundational necessity for the act of living. Balance has become so critical to healthy living, that society is quick to hospitalize those with severe balance issues, for their own safety. **Society has determined that people with severe balance issues, are not capable of safe independent living.**

Balance, as taught by Shashi yoga, covers areas not covered by most other yoga styles with limited movements or limited positions, in fact balance is so important to our health and independence, Shashi spends a lot of time teaching balance in his classes, balance is a major element in one's education in yoga.

"We think we are so smart," Shashi says time and again. "We may be intelligent, but we aren't smart." Shashi also says, "If we were smart, we would take better care of our bodies."

Time is a poor excuse for not taking care of our bodies— we should make time.

Maintaining Balance

Shashi Yoga has dozens of balance tests and exercises and a wealth of knowledge in balance. Only by regular practice can we maintain our balancing abilities and expand on them.

Balance is a sister to Grounding, as you might recall in chapter eight (8) and they work together. While balance and yoga help to shape and mold the body. Grounding, gives roots and taps the earth's Life Force and stabilizes the body.

Pain killers, blood pressure medications and other drugs the doctor prescribes plays havoc with our balance, topped with the weakening of our legs, feet and toes as we use them less.

If you believe that any of your medications are affecting your balance negatively, ask your doctor if he/she has another medication that wouldn't affect your balance. Meanwhile, be more careful that you don't fall and practice your balancing exercises more and practice your leg and toe strengthening exercises more. **For heavens sake, If your doctor tells you to use a cane for safety, then Do it!**

Life's Gift

I can't close this chapter on balance without talking about what one might expect from life when total balance is achieved.

Yes… **"Life's Gift"** Earlier, I told you of an interview Shashi once gave. The interviewer asked Shashi, *"what he wanted most"*? Shashi said, that *"he wanted most to make his students enlightened"*. Shashi is excited to have the gift of seeing aura's and he is excited to be able to teach and give lessons in yoga that he loves so much.

I understand that when the body is in total balance, we receive the purity of a child's view (viewing great wonders from the heart), **that there is a gift for each of us.** My parents are of European and Gaelic heritage, the wonders of children's *fairy tales* filled my childhood. Magical Birds, Golden Eggs, Leprechauns, Rainbow Bridges. Including the Happiest of song and dance music.

With a child's perception we can see "Truth". That our garden is not just a garden, that our garden is a Magical Garden. That the ocean is not just an Ocean, but a Magical Sea filled with many wonders.

Yoga has a lot to give. Besides the Wonderful Gifts of better health, **life has a gift for each of us.** What do you think your gift is, or will be?

CHAPTER 11

BABY STEPS

Why "Baby Steps" in yoga? Shashi observed, not all beginning students of yoga are of equal health and flexibility. Not all students have the same occupation, nor are they all the same age.

Seeing students progress and seeing their health improve is so pleasing to Shashi, that he honestly feels that his students' bodies send him their blessings.

"Baby Steps" in yoga may sound like something of such little value, that one might think to one self that it would be better to wait until one felt better, or stronger…We think, "Then I'll start on a stronger foot". **Not a good idea!**

For example: After surgery, a doctor knows the importance of therapy and that first step. **Doctors get the patient up almost immediately after surgery.**

Athletes may not mention the words "Baby Steps" for any of their workouts. However, what these athletes call "warm-up exercises," are pretty much "Baby Steps," compared to the event that these athletes are warming up for. No one should be embarrassed by "Baby Steps."

We are all familiar with the story of the race between the rabbit and the turtle and how the turtle won the race. Slow and steady adds up. We should never underestimate the progress one can make with small steps.

Full speed in life isn't always practical. High speeds in life, as unknown roads and highways are good examples of Life's unknown situations, where no one should feel embarrassed at slowing down or taking "Baby Steps".

One of the lessons of a good yoga teacher, school, or studio, is not to let our egos bully us into abandoning logic.

Shashi has a mantra he teaches his students when they feel that their mind is not acting logically. Shashi says, When our mind chatters illogically, that we should tell the mind… "Shut-up."

We have all known people who let their Ego get in their way. Don't be ashamed of small steps; "Baby Steps" add up.

Johnny Appleseed

In early American history, a man traveling west planted apples along the way and became known as Johnny Appleseed. The amount of trees Johnny planted that survived was phenomenal. One day the "Baby Steps" we take today may grow into trees of knowledge and fantastic health.

One day the "Baby Steps" that we plant today may grow into trees of knowledge and fantastic health. These trees of knowledge and experience may not benefit only us, but others as well. Like the seeds planted by Johnny Apple Seed, not only spreading beauty as he "walked" west, the trees grew. It's said that Johnny's trees later gave wonderful fruit.

People in Johnny Appleseed's day laughed at Johnny and called him crazy, but Johnny didn't care.

I like to think of Johnny Appleseed as an early American Yogi.

Apples, like yoga have been found to be very good for the health. A slogan has even been written regarding apples, you might remember, that states, "an apple a day keeps the doctor away."

Small doesn't always mean low in value.

Science and movement

Shashi is always sharing some of his knowledge of science. Often, he shares Amazing facts, like the short life of cells and despite their short lives, they pass on all their knowledge before they die.

Fear of not being the most flexible person in the room is no reason to deny one's body some precious movements, even when we can only move our bodies with "Baby Steps". Our wonderful bodies need movement. The body's pharmaceutical and chemical plants, as well as the various energy fields created by movement are many and all are important.

We must be our own accountant and balance our body's energy finances and determine, how we should invest or spend our life Force Energies.

Modern science is still trying to duplicate many of the chemicals and energies created by movement that we can only perceive as heat. The rivers of electrical energy that flows from the furthermost parts of our bodies, from head to toe, are not to be regarded as anything less than fantastic. The Ancients knew a lot about the body and yoga that modern day science is only now confirming with research and documentation.

Yoga Dividends

When normal chores seem difficult, we should recognize that the body needs both Attention and Time, often the body really needs several hours of yoga. Compared to the probable need of several hours of yoga, that our bodies could sure use to fix the body, that amount is quite small in comparison to the length of time we abused our bodies.

Shashi Yoga is so structured and well-managed like a professional investment portfolio. Where our bodies and minds receive dividends from both ancient yoga and modern science, from just one hour a day practice at home. Shashi Yoga is like two sound Blue Chip, Mutual Funds (to speak of) that of science and that of yoga. Both have a history of giving health and hope and continue to give health and hope dividends.

Tremendous results are even reported by people who have only **invested minutes** a day. Now that's real progress from real small, "Baby Steps!"

When I first started taking Shashi Yoga, my practice habits weren't very good and I had not yet acquired much faith in Shashi Yoga. I started receiving compliments from my doctor and other people, even before I noticed any improvement. Small steps may seem like hardly anything …but they do pay off.

CHAPTER 12

FEET AND HANDS

Our Base and Our Potential

Two amazing subjects Feet (our Base) and Hands (our Potential). *Our feet* can carry us great distances and great heights, in the direction of our potential. Our *hands* can mold, create, build and even help a child, a neighbor, or help an animal.

Although our Base is not always the feet, in yoga our Base can be sitting or lying as well, *this chapter is on the feet and hands,* Balance is so critical and so neglected in life, in this chapter I refer almost totally to our Base as our feet, since we are on our feet so much. Shashi strives to enhance all the elements necessary for a strong, flexible, healthy Base, no matter where that base might be., so that our feet can be all that they can be. (as I use the Army moto "Be all that you can be").

Feet, Shashi goes to great lengths to impress upon his students the importance of the foundation of the body. The foundation of the body is sometimes called, "the base".

Shashi often compares the foundation of the body to the foundation of a building, needing a good foundation. Students are encouraged to memorize the number of bones, muscles and pressure points in the feet, which is 28 bones and 33 muscles and 52 pressure points in the feet.

The base, the foundation, the root, determine the strength of a structure.

Some health-related fields minimize the role of the feet, even to the point of omitting (from their schools, or classes) any mention of the feet being important, nor the important role feet play in balance.

The root structure, determines the strength and health of a plant or tree. Seldom do we think about the fact, that the root is the "Heart" of a tree or plant and is fed directly by the mother earth, receiving directly the mother earth's "Life Force" *as she wraps so lovingly the roots, with the earth/ soil* **(Mother Earth's version of the water of the womb). Little do we realize the sacredness of our feet, which dwell in the aura of Mother earth.**

The Animals, from which science says mankind has evolved, usually have four feet. Having four feet provides a wider, stronger base than man has with only two legs, providing another lesson for us in yoga, a wider base provides us more strength, stability and much better balance.

Separating one's feet not only provides better balance, it changes both the foundation and the balance. Like a tree extending their roots not only deep but wide. Roots anchoring the plant or tree, to rocks, soil and adobe provides even more stability and taps an even wider range of earth's frequencies.

We should never view our feet as anything less than a **second heart**, never neglecting nor abusing them and by all means we should never take our feet for granted. Thousands of people have lost their feet and were unable to adjust to prosthetics and had to go to rest homes.

Shashi always talks about how the nerves in the body spans the entire body, not only from head to toe but extend to the fingers and toes as well. Science, as well as Shashi acknowledges the existence of pressure points that affect the body and even extend into both the hands and feet.

Those of us in yoga need to ground our lives to rock solid good health practices, one of which is Shashi's advised practice of *mindful movement with the breath.* Our entire bodies are still wired as if we were still walking on all four feet. **We are going against the body's design when we don't move our arms when we walk or run, as our shoulders and hips are still wired to work together, as the last day man ran on all four.**

The Army has known for centuries the need to move the body as though the body's limbs were a second heart. We were told: "Pump those arms!", "Pump those legs!"

Many people in yoga, at one time in their life, have studied martial arts. Shashi has had such a background and has brought a lesson from martial arts to yoga. The lesson is that in war or fights, the placing of the feet widely apart provides more stability and balance, as the body (feet) is more anchored to the ground, then as the knees are slightly bent and bending slightly at the waist, one is in a position that in martial arts is called "The Horse". **As the martial artist assumes "The Horse" position they are assuming the most stable balance position he/she can assume, as they wait for the unexpected.**

In yoga we learn our balance is better with our feet apart and still better a little further apart. As mathematical rules apply in construction, with the placing of studs for the walls, there are rules for the best position of the feet, such as, that it is best not to spread one's feet further than *shoulder width*, in most cases for balance while standing.

Shashi Yoga also gives more information on learning to diagnose the body's need for positioning the feet. On uphill slopes, we see a need for strong toes and a need to lean forward. On downhill slopes, we dig our heals in and lean back. Shashi teaches balance for different situations.

Mindfully Positioning the Feet

My father was involved in high-rise construction for a while, I understand. People in high-rise construction know the importance of a strong, solid base. These people in high-rise construction really have to know about foundations and the ground where they plan to build. The ground determines so much about the foundation of the building they propose to build. For example, sand is so unstable, special measures need to be taken for stabilization of a project, where the area they plan to build is largely sand.

Foundations are important in the Building Trade however the importance of needed studies are really magnified with high-rise buildings foundations. So many studies are needed in the preparation and construction of high-rise buildings foundations. Foundations must allow for the proper distribution of weight.

We should mindfully prepare our feet as an architect would prepare the plans, for a building they propose to build. We owe our bodies and our feet the very best care and attention that we can possibly give, as we prepare our bodies for exceptionally good health.

Connection to the Higher Brain

As we practice our yoga, learn and update on a regular basis, we strengthen the body and expand our minds.

With our bodies healthy and our brains strengthened, we approach the grand prize of yoga, "The Higher Brain". A frequency of consciousness beyond the physical.

I had an uncle who had an accident as a child. He was unable to move his arms and had no control of his hands. My uncle Erv (short for Ervin), developed the ability to use his feet so well that, if you dropped a coin on the floor, he could pick it up faster with his feet than we could with our hands. My uncle Erv could smoke cigars with his feet, play cards, eat and sign his checks with his feet. I've seen the power of the feet that modern man has lost.

What power a healthy person would possess who developed long lost abilities, along with regular moving abilities. Like the ability to have the sensitive hearing and touch that the blind possesses. These lost senses reactivated could trigger great accomplishments in human evolution.

Health is so precious we shouldn't wait until we lose it before we explore the wonders of the body and the wonders of yoga. Why must we wait until we have a tragic event in our lives, before we explore our existing abilities and how to replace lost abilities or lost health, due to sickness or accidents?

Today, we are so blessed to have been born in this "Spring Time of Wonder", that our hands and feet, like children can play and take part in the miracles of the budding and blooming, advancing technologies and love. Shashi Yoga is One of the gorgeous flowers in this "Spring Time of Wonder" for maintaining our bodies (We can learn Shashi Yoga and enjoy this season of "Wonder").

Hands and the Mind

Hands, created by the designer of our bodies. What a fantastic creation! **By the Hands we know so much about the mind**, Sincerity, Kindness, Strength, Love, Maturity, Sex, Confidence, even one's interest in Music and Dance. Our hands reveal a lot about us.

Like our bodies our Hands receive so little credit and attention for the wonders that they perform. Old pictures show *Divine Hands* as in "The Creation". What better way to depict "Creation", than with Hands of Age, Hands or Strength, Hands of Wisdom, Hands of Power, Hands that can lift a fallen Tree, or Hold a Flower, or a Butterfly?

As Humans were given the gift of a Body, a Mind and Hands, **we were also given, the "*Science of Yoga*" to Maintain our Body's, our Minds and our Hands.** We were also given the ability to teach our children the "*Science of Yoga*", that they could either accept or reject yoga for their lives.

Hands are such a piece of work, that they boggle the mind for mankind's capabilities of coordinating the mind and the hands. No wonder we have become enormously dependent on the hands; for our very survival is linked to our hands which feed entertain and protect us as well.

We learn in yoga that the brain connects every part of the body. Even now, science is confirming that not only does the brain control the body, the body also affects the brain.

Shashi has a lot of respect for acupressure and acupuncture as both fields chart parts of the body being connected to the hands and feet. In Shashi Yoga we are taught how nerves from our toes to our fingers connect to our brains.

Shashi Yoga teaches stretches with hand positions allowing us to stretch our bodies in more ways and use more muscles, that allow a far better strength distribution and balance for our body's strength.

Shashi teaches how hand positions affect different parts of the lungs during breathing exercises, that placing the hands above the heart during breathing exercises affect different (seldom used) lobes of the lungs and that in India, it is believed that shaking the fingers of the hands, while swinging the arms in giant circles with the elbows straight, is said to make one happy.

CHAPTER 13

TOOLS

The Cost of Comfort

"Tools," was the first lecture I remember Shashi giving when I started taking classes. I seemed to understand the need for Shashi Yoga. Why wasn't I told this in school? It was sure different, but it made sense!

Beds, are so soft Shashi explained, that they bend our spines in several places for hours as we sleep, molding our spines and internal organs into unhealthy positions and that it is not good either for our joints to be molded into those positions nor the unhealthy position that our joints are put in. Beauty experts tell us that how we sleep and our habits wrinkles our skin (our largest organ) then imagine the damage created inside our bodies from un healthy positions in bed.

Chairs, we learn are of such a height that over time the leg muscles would grow so weak that after a few years, when we attempt a sitting or squatting position just below the chair's seat level, these lower positions become almost impossible to attain.

Over-Stuffed Chairs, are great to sit in when we are healthy. But for the old or sick, when they attempt to get up, these over-stuffed chairs become like a trap. The old or the sick need help to escape from the chair that has them in its clutches.

Shoes, are not healthy to wear all the time, sure our feet need protection *at times*, but they also **need to "feel"** the ground, **to**

deny our feet the ability to "feel" is a terrible thing to do to our feet, it is a terrible thing to do to our toes and our balance (imagine if we were not allowed to give our fingers their complete range of motion that they need?). Every day when we put on our shoes, we are putting 28 bones, 33 muscles and 52 pressure points in what amounts to be coffins. To constantly wear shoes **is to impose a death sentence to our feet our balance and our bodies.**

Comfort, like candy or some kind of drug, the hope or promise of comfort can be so inviting, so tempting that we over do, over indulge, in that fabulous drug we call comfort. We think we are so smart! As we allow comfort to take a more and more prominent role in our lives, we search for more and more tools, just so we can do less and less. Telling ourselves that we are tired. When we are *actually lazy.*

Challenges of Technology

Cars, have been the cause of us walking less and less, we have gotten in such a habit of taking the car for extremely short distances that we very well could have walked.

Cell Phones, are needed for work and our personal lives. This is another "Tool" that brings health issues. Wither the health issue stems from radiation, neck position (text Neck), dexterity (carpal tunnel), or mental laziness. As these challenges and changes take place, we should try and be prepared. Shashi Yoga has therapy exercises for "Text Neck" and "Carpal Tunnel" that help us keep up with both challenges and changes.

Computers, of course brought big changes both in the home and the work place, "Repetitive Stress Symptoms" was exceptionally rampant in the work place. Shashi was hired by a prominent corporation to create computer stations, some of which allowed standing. This helped a lot in the workplace, also showing the respect Shashi enjoys with his background of yoga and the human body. At Shashi's yoga school, success was and is still greater.

Life is just doing its thing, providing constant Challenges, Constant Changes. Again, there is an appropriate quote from Shashi dealing with coping with Life's Changes and Challenges. "We think we are so smart, but we are not… we are only intelligent". We need to be smarter and above all, we need a tool called "Wisdom", located in the "Higher Brain".

Is it worth sleeping in a feather bed, with pillows placed here and there for additional comfort, knowing full well that due to this tool of temporary comfort we are actually harming our bodies? We are actually laying the groundwork for many years of health issues, such as problems with the spine, joints, shoulders, hips, neck and more.

As a child I do recall a popular saying, **"If you want to dance, you have to pay the fiddler."** (If you stayed up late, you would miss-out on a good night's sleep. If you drank a lot of alcohol you might get sick or have a head ache in the morning, if you over eat, again you might get sick or have a stomach ache. **There is a cost to Body Abuse!**)

Shashi uses a saying a lot, that was a very popular saying when I was a kid. "If you can't fix it, Don't Break it!" (Referring to the difficulty to Fix the body)

Like a skill saw we are using at home or, in our work shop that may have a warning sticker. **There should be a warning sticker on life, "Warning Life can be Dangerous".**

The Science of Self-Healing

Have we become so spoiled that we give up to quickly? We have heard so many horror stories on TV, In the News, at School, we run to quickly to the doctor these days. We don't know the difference in discomfort and pain, or soreness and pain.

We have become so spoiled, that we cook for ourselves less and less, we hardly wash our own clothes, hardly do our own cleaning, we seldom do our own gardening, nor do we make our own music. **We don't trust our own thinking...**we use calculators to do our math. The fact that we go to the tv to tell us how to vote… is sad. **But we "give up" to soon on our "Bodies Self-Healing Abilities" and "Yoga's Prevention Abilities".**

Is it in fact that we are "lazy" and expect God or doctors to heal us instantly? Or do we "bail-out" of our duties in life and die escaping to heaven? Or do we want to die early (escaping our duties) expecting a reincarnation "where life is a bed of roses".

The longer we do yoga, the better the chance is that besides gaining good health, the better the chance we will be able to deal with life's challenges with our "Higher Brain".

CHAPTER 14

STRETCHING

The Controlled Stretch

As with any Shashi Yoga "Mindful movement with the breath", is the Shashi Yoga way.

All body movements in yoga requires Mindfulness, in this controlled stretch we mindfully dissect the art of the stretch with an imaginary demonstrator.

Let's assume that we have an imaginary demonstrator. This imaginary demonstrator has climbed a fruit tree and while standing on a thick, secure branch, our demonstrator chooses to pick a piece of fruit, as He / She reaches for this piece of fruit with their right hand, they are holding onto a secure limb, above their head with their left hand.

It's good that we visualize "The Anatomy of The Stretch".

Focusing

The Demonstrator "Focuses" on the piece of fruit that they want to pick. Determining the distance and the science of the stretch, the placement of the feet and how much the body needs to lean into the stretch (possible body adjustments, like leaning).

Awareness

Our demonstrator exercises their awareness, determining their location in relation to the fruit and if it is a safe stretch or not? Is the fruit worth the stretch? Meanwhile, our demonstrator is aware of their own balance and of their own comfort in that position.

Speed

Our demonstrator determines a speed for the stretch (reach) and if additional body adjustments is necessary to reach the piece of fruit they chose to pick.

Hold Time

Hold Time, is the time it takes our demonstrator to pull, twist, or pick that piece of fruit, from the stem holding it.

Retraction Design (Plan)

Mentally Designing the release of the stretch, balance is considered, as well as the return route and possible stages of movement and speed, while maintaining awareness.

Retraction (acting upon the plan)

From the start to finish of the retraction, the release of the stretch begins as planned, always aware of needed changes in speed, stages of movement and movement adjustments,

Thanks to our imaginary demonstrator, we have learned that the "Anatomy of The Stretch" consists of six (6) steps.

1) **Focusing,** on the stretch.
2) **Awareness,** the detail

3) **Speed** and possible body adjustments.
4) **Hold Time**
5) **Retraction (plan)**

6) **Retraction (Act)**

Even an action which seems as simple as a "Stretch" needs us to act from the state of mind, that Shashi refers to as "Mindfulness".

Benefits of A Stretch

Every muscle, every part of the body needs to stretch. To "Stretch", we already know that in essence To Stretch, is to **"Reach For!"**

"To Stretch" is to **"Reach For"**

We started this chapter with an imaginary demonstrator, who demonstrated an imaginary stretch for an imaginary piece of fruit, in our "Anatomy of A Stretch".

The "Anatomy of A Stretch" as depicted above can also depict the crying out of the body, as the body *must* **"Reach For"** the body's needs.

To feed our body's Needs. (We must "Stretch" as a parent would "Reach" for their child's needs).

One: We must "Stretch" our bodies for the needed **Blood / Circulation** it will receive, by **"Reaching For"**.

Two: We must "Stretch" our bodies for the needed **Oxygen** it will receive, by **"Reaching For"**.

Three: We must "Stretch" our bodies for the needed **Strength** it will receive by **"Reaching For"**.

Four: We must "Stretch" our bodies for the needed **Flexibility** it will receive by **"Reaching For"**.

If we start "Stretching" while we are healthy, just the act of "Reaching For" and a little time with the Science of Yoga "The Cookie Jar of Health" (will make our life a lot sweeter).

Cautions

Check with your Doctor, Physical Therapist, Yoga Instructor, or Personal Trainer before doing Stretches seen on TV, the Internet, or in Magazines, or recommended by non-professional friends.

Professional Athletes require stretches and exercises close to the type of movement in their sport. **General stretches** are often recommended to be *avoided* before their events, as they often cause an athlete not to do as well in that event.

The General public is usually advised to stretch only the larger muscle masses with-out a professionals' guidance.

CHAPTER 15

THE SPINE

Shashi's Entire Body Approach

Even science talks about the "Spine" being like a telephone switchboard because of all the nerves from all over the body in the spine.

Scientific findings have now determined that the spine is a switchboard for the body's nerve endings, this proves Shashi's teachings are right, that the entire body is connected and needs to be viewed, as the "Total Being" that it is. Shashi has said for years that aches and pains in the arm or leg does not mean that the arm or leg was the origin of the problem causing the pain in the arm or leg.

Shashi's teachings that treatments for the body's ailments should cover the entire body, that with the spine rerouting signals at the switchboard of the spine, a problem could very well have originated in any number of places in the body.

Records of China's Ancient Warriors, who were shot with arrows document, that the arrow's wounds affected other parts of the body, often some distance from the arrows' wound. In fact, the records are documented so well, that this is said to be how the foundation of acupuncture and acupressure was established.

Shashi says that as a youth, he was a "Yoga Demonstrator" in India along with *a very flex able cousin*. **By careful observation we can learn a lot from a demonstrator.** As we view a demonstrator (since this chapter is on the "Spine", we might particularly take mental notes of the demonstrator's attention to the Spine). A demonstrator is a shinning example of how important the proper technique is, for the information that is to be conveyed to the audience. Regarding the demonstrator and the Spine: Let me tell you some of the things the demonstrator may be trying to convey to the audience. **The vertebrae in the neck are said to be the weakest of the vertebrae, one reason perhaps that Shashi suggests, that we don't stand on our heads.**

Sudden jerking movements while twisting or turning the body can cause "Hyper Extension" of the muscles, a form of rupture of a joint. Shashi's "Mindful Movement with the Breath" does a lot to help regulate the speed and safety of the movement, causing a more fluid movement for the exercise.

The Spine is a perfect example of Shashi's, whole body approach to maintaining, as well as fixing the body. I am sure, the spine's massive amount of nerves and the muscles, even in the proximity of the spine, could make diagnosing of a pain quite challenging, for the most experienced doctors.

I was told years ago by a karate instructor, that the body is designed as it is to protect the "Spine." The "Spine" he said, was placed behind us "so that it is protected", that the spine "was special: a prize."

In that form, the martial artist had a technique to spin his opponent around and disable his opponent and attack his opponent's spine. Or to stun his opponent and then to attack his opponent's spine. No drawn-out fighting! The longer the fight, the more chance your opponent could get lucky and kill you.

Making Our Health Our Hobby

Since we are discussing the "Spine" in this chapter and the Spine has within its' domain, ties to the entire body.

Often when Shashi is talking about Science and Yoga, he will say with our utmost well-being in mind, as he often says to verify a point "Ask a good scientist, or better yet make science your hobby."

Perhaps we should take Shashi's suggestion and make Science together with Yoga and our Health, our Hobby?

Shashi Yoga would be an excellent way to start a "Hobby" with educating ourselves and installing a habit of "Mindful Movement with the Breath."

Our spines deserve a lot more respect than they get. The spine is so strong, so flexible. With powers so great, I wonder how many of the myths are true about the metaphysical powers of the spine. What ever your interest, if you have an interest in Metaphysics, Science, Health, The Higher Brain, or Religious ideas, then explore those ideas along with Yoga for an added incentive to do Yoga and take your well-being to heights that you never imagined.

We must realize that "Life" is an "Elevator of Results." That for every action or lack of action there will be an up or down movement in our lives.

Evolution of the Spine

Science says that by the looks of our tailbones that humans once had tails. Shashi even has exercises where if we had tails, their movement and balance could benefit both the body and the brain.

Although we don't have tails, the exercise seems beneficial to the spine hips and intestines.

Scientists say that we use our little toes so seldom that they expect us to eventually lose our little toes through evolution.

If we did have tails and eventually lost them through evolution, I wonder how they would have affected our brains and our potential? If every limb, every appendage, connects to our brains and if a potential exists in our minds because of these limbs and appendages, then, what potential did we lose in our brains when we lost our tails?

We are capable of multiple actions at the same time, due to multiple limbs and appendages. Perhaps as each finger on a hand strengthens the hand and each toe on a foot strengthens the foot and our second eye strengthens our sight. Two arms, most definitely increases our lifting ability over one. Two legs are the minimum of legs necessary for walking.

Although a tail's contribution to the brain is questionable… Shashi is concerned that technology has reached a point where young people are using their minds less and less, raising concerns, even fears of minds and bodies atrophying. If the mind atrophies to a point of loss of mental abilities, as the body is losing its abilities and balance, Shashi is concerned and wants to help.

Recently While dinning with some friends, I over-heard the question asked, "Why a lizard's tail continued to wiggle, although the tail was detached from the lizard?

The answer astounded me. The reply was, *that the lizard had a "Second Brain in the Tail",* That the lizard's second brain would cause the detached tail to continue to wiggle to confuse the lizard's enemy and that the lizard could get away and would grow a new tail.

Wow! I had never heard of a second brain in the tail. If humans ever had a second brain in their tails, that could have been a sizeable loss for humans. A second brain could possibly help explain some of the unexplained mysteries of ancient man's intelligence.

Shashi talks a lot about **"Text Neck"** (a condition caused by people hunched over, looking at their electronic devices for hours at a time that it puts an extreme load on the spine).

To be as accurate as possible about "Text Neck," I checked the internet and found an article published in the journal, "Surgical Technology International" and it is quoted

as showing that when you are standing or sitting straight your head weighs 10 to 12 lbs. on average. But if you lean 15 degrees forward, the heads' weight is more like 27 lbs. With a 30 degree tilt the weight is more like 40 lbs.

Studying without a Teacher

Studying yoga without a certified yoga teacher can be "Dangerous", even when traveling in India. Shashi says there are so many unlicensed people in India who force their students into positions that cause serious injuries all the time.

California has a wonderful requirement for teachers to have a minimum of 200 hours of training and an insurance requirement for the safety of their students.

Since this chapter is on "The Spine," Here are some of the reasons to be cautious with the treatment of the spine, as Spinal Cord injuries can not only cause severe **injuries,** but spinal cord injuries can even cause **death.**

Spinal Cord Injury: When tears occur in the ligaments the vertebrae may slip out of normal alignment and the spinal cord may be injured.

Muscle Injury: Whiplash can cause injuries of the neck muscles, ranging from minor strains and microhemorrhages to severe tears.

Whiplash Injuries of the Head and Neck: Whiplash injuries of the head and neck is caused by a sudden exaggerated thrust of the head backwards, forwards, and sometimes sideways.

Hyperextension: When the head is forced backward in hyperextension, pieces of bone may be pulled from cervical vertebrae by a tear of the anterior longitudinal ligament. Spinous processes of the vertebrae may be fractured.

Hyperflexion: The head is propelled in a forward and downward motion in hyperflexion. Possibly crushing an anterior portion of vertebrae.

Spinal Ligaments: In a whiplash injury, ligaments may be badly stretched, partially torn, or completely ruptured.

Ligament Damage: Anterior longitudinal ligaments, running vertically along the anterior surface of the vertebrae may be injured during hyperextension. The posterior longitudinal ligament, running on the posterior surface of the vertebral bodies, may be injured in hyperflexion.

The Life Force

"Mindful Movement with the Breath." How wonderful that Shashi bases his teachings on the fantastic concept of, "Mindful Movement with the Breath," this is the concept that I was taught long ago for *Recognizing* and '*the Beginning* of working with the "Life Force".

Some of the goals of Shashi Yoga, I understand are, besides Great Health, is accessing the Higher Brain, with eventual enlightenment, as results of balancing the body and the mind with Scientifically designed exercises and "Mindful Movement with the Breath".

Although In the beginning one may feel that they are just feeling the blood in the area of their attention… and perhaps they are…**Yet, when this "Blood is Oxygenated by the Breath," now, it ceases to be "just blood." Besides the Blood and the Oxygen supplied by the Breath; The World's Greatest Pharmaceutical Factory has already determined the body's needs of medicines, some still unknown to modern medicine, is passed into this oxygenated fluid that we call blood. This "Blood" is now Energized, Medicated and Oxygenated, in reality it has become much more than mere "Blood."**

What-ever you excel at or do well, where time magically disappears, into what you are doing, weather it is Art, Sports, Business, it is because **you are putting your life force into it** that you do so well.

As You Breath, your energy, your "Life Force" passes into your mindful movement **"Feeling"** is a major key. Seeing energy is great but we must **"Feel"** to **know the power and to be able to control the force.**

Like fingers together give strength to the hand. Sticks, or even straws tied together, make a bundle extremely strong.

There are pictures of different colored lines coiling upward in yoga or metaphysical books, representing different energies. In yoga, we learn to see beauty and experience the joy we "Feel" in our Life Force, as we do yoga or meditate. By all means learn to "Feel" and see the joy of other "Life Forces" in nature. Rather than dwelling on fear and discomfort in life.

Shashi Yoga doesn't talk about the use of the "Life Force" energies in class, Shashi talks about Science and "Mindful Movement with the Breath". Shashi talks about the body healing it-self, maintaining it-self. Shashi talks about doing Yoga and Meditation at home.

As we become Mindful of our Bodies and our Breath, we will find that Mindfulness is a tuning devise in the Radio of the Higher Brain, for detecting and later befriending these frequencies and "Forces of Nature".

Many of you have studied the power of the Kundalini in yoga and Meditation. Many of you have studied the power of the Chi in martial arts. Although, Shashi Yoga is a soft form of maintaining the body. I like to point out that by working with "Mindful Movement with the Breath," as Shashi teaches. **Unbelievable benefits still exist in Shashi Yoga, even though Shashi doesn't promote the benefits of the "Life Force", Shashi does promote the world's greatest Physician that is within our bodies and the world's greatest pharmacy, that also resides in our bodies.** Shashi Yoga, it does seem that if followed to the letter, can take the student to the "Higher Brain."

CHAPTER 16

INTERNAL ORGANS

Internal Organs, their function and their maintenance are so-o Fascinating, Mesmerizing even Enchanting when studying the human body. The wisdom, grace and beauty of the body's use of water, air (breath), movement, diet, sight and sound, can charm an investigating student like an Enchanting Mysterious woman.

Each Subject has drawn the greatest minds the world has ever known to chase those subjects and win their secrets.

Presently, Shashi Yoga has captured many of these mysterious Subjects secrets. The fragrance of these reviled wisdom secrets, fills Shashi Yoga like a love story.

Shashi Yoga does have the perfumed fragrance of wisdom by Maintaining the inside of the body *before* we have internal problems and using sound frequencies for inside the brain provides not only much needed therapeutic vibrations for the brain, but the body as well. Sound also aids other delicate areas like inside and behind the eyes, not accessible by any other means.

While doing some exercises, Shashi might explain which organs are affected by the exercise, the organ's function and the organs needs.

Shashi also teaches mistaken concepts regarding the heart and seldom taught facts about how necessary the lungs' role is for the heart to function well. Another heart concern by many is that the heart is only one and the only organ of its type in the body. However, we learn in Shashi Yoga that the diaphragm can be used with the breath, as a pump which helps to soften the heart's work load.

Besides explaining the exercises in his classes, Shashi also explains how exercise practices once thought beneficial for maintaining our health, are not as beneficial as they were once thought to be. **Actually, practices like running treadmills, swimming and more, are really so often using the body not fixing the body.**

Besides the heart, Shashi talks a lot about the stomach, that we should not over eat, that the stomach cavity has so many important organs that need space and our attention. Shashi is always promoting "Mindful Movement with the breath" which is a "must" in repairing, "fixing" Shashi's term for repairing the body.

After a lot of breathing exercises, Shashi has his students blow out any remaining air, then hold their breath briefly and to move their stomach.

Notice, Shashi's attention to the body's internal need of movement.

Shashi teaches his exercises Sitting, Standing and even some laying down as different positions affect the breath and different mussels. For example, we learn when doing breathing exercises, that our arm positions above the heart, uses different lobes of the lungs. For those interested in walking, Shashi loves teaching what he calls the "Yogi Walk."

Shashi also teaches an almost snoring type of breath, that he calls "OOU-JAY" and different vowel sounds with the breath, while exhaling. These techniques I understand, are good for the throat and good for controlling the breath, it is said that making the vowels sounds, when exhaling, have multiple benefits, such as creating calming and healing frequencies. It is important to see the attention to detail that Shashi pays to updating yoga.

Shashi explains that so many students ask for training in meditation, yet can't sit still for five minutes. These people need to practice yoga first so they can learn to quiet the mind, or they are wasting their money.

In Shashi Yoga, not only are there exercises to benefit the body; In Shashi's classes, he also explains how the exercises help, the mind, limbs and the internal organs. In Shashi's classes he also explains how his exercises **help the many systems** in the body: Like the Skeletal, Muscular, Lymph, Glandular, Nervous and Circulatory systems. **A far cry from merely concentrating on the flexibility of the body, as so many yoga studios do.** We must give credit to Shashi Yoga for the vastness or scope of benefits that it brings, to those who practice Shashi Yoga.

Any practice claiming to benefit humanity or claiming the title of "Yoga," must adhere to or stick to what yoga stands for: "union of body, mind and spirit."

Shashi Yoga targets the body's and the mind's *needs*, allowing for a healthier body. So, one can pursue their goals with a healthier body, withier their goals are athletic, or spiritual goals, the yoga practitioner will be more physically and mentally prepared and if the yoga practitioner's goals are spiritual, Shashi Yoga has students from all the major religions of the world. With so many religious students taking Shashi Yoga classes, proves Shashi Yoga is effective for students in pursuit of spiritual goals, as well as physical health pursuits.

Shashi Yoga doesn't just teach Body "Needs," such as Balance, Strength and Agility, *nor does he stop* at adding a wealth of information on the Breath. Shashi Yoga, teaches us about the Pharmaceutical Factories of, our body's Endocrine System, their locations and exercises to keep these Glands (The controllers of our body's functions) healthy.

The Endocrine glands through the use of creating needed chemicals for the body, is one of the pharmaceutical factories in the body that Shashi marvels at.

The Endocrine glands, Shashi explains, is actually a "System" infusing **custom chemicals** directly into the blood "Targeting" the needs of the body's operating system, which includes hormones that regulate, metabolism, growth and development, tissue function, sexual function, reproduction, sleep and the body's range of moods and more. **Here are the Five (5) Glands listed in the Endocrine System: The Pineal Gland, The Adrenal Gland, The Thyroid Gland, The Thymus Gland and The Prostate Gland.**

If you haven't tried Shashi Yoga, maybe you should try it, even if you need to go out of your way, your health is worth it.

When I was a child, my parents read to me a story of a magic golden Apple. Reach for it! Shashi Yoga can be **"Your Golden Apple"** of good health. Polish your yoga skills every day. Good Health is a treasure.

True, Shashi Yoga isn't in every city yet! Also, to get the best results one needs to put some time in, at home, for the best results. But just between you and me...you will be happiest with what you have to reach for! "Stretch For," **those apples we stretch for, are usually the "Most-Tasty."**

CHAPTER 17

JOINTS & SPACE

Hopefully you know by now, that Shashi continually talks about, *"mindful movement with the breath."* No book or article about Shashi Yoga could ever be written about Shashi Yoga that doesn't mention, *"Mindful movement with the breath."*

This entire book is my attempt (a lay person) to give a view of Shashi Yoga that average people can understand. So, in my attempt to not be too repetitious, I have not used Shashi's phrase of *"mindful movement with the breath,"* enough in other chapters.

We need to be especially mindful of the art of movement in this chapter. As this chapter deals with the hinges and rotary hardware of life, (the hinges and rotary joints).

In Shashi's classes, he describes the anatomy of the joints, the restrictions of the hinge and rotary joints and both the healthy and the unhealthy (arthritic) joints.

Shashi explains the danger of omitting seemingly simplistic exercises of the wrist, with these exercises **it is important that the student can safely bend their wrist at a 45-degree angle to the arm** in order to support their weight safely, to prevent injury. Shashi further explains that a student who can't bend their wrist safely at a 45-degree angle to the arm, then it would not be safe for the student to do some floor exercises safely without possible injury.

Shashi cautions his students, that we should never put weight on a joint that we can't bend.

Space as mentioned in the title of this chapter, space is very much a needed element, in the equation of movement. Space, mentioned here in the title of this chapter, is referring to the space needed, in our joints for our smooth, fluid, movements and for healthy joints of the body.

I wonder if this fantastic subject of space in the human body is available in books for non-medical or non-scientifically employed people?

Space is often discussed in Shashi's lectures on the body. Besides, the joints need of space in the Joints, space is also a needed element in the process of digestion. Like the body's need of air, water and food, **"Space" is essential for a healthy functioning body.**

Formulas in the science of yoga appear everywhere I turn. As Shashi explains, that we should have the proper ratio of space to water and food in the digestive system, while acids break down the food and create gasses.

Inner and Outer Space

Discussions and lectures on space, both inner and outer space, all make me think of the sci-fi movies and the fantastic phrase, "Space...The Last Frontier," "The Great unknown." All so true! There is so much we can learn from space. Like untold secrets, unknown sciences, and unseen powers and un-explored energy fields.

In yoga, we learn of the powers of the "unseen," like Atoms, Prana, the Breath, Sunlight, Darkness, Electricity and Gravity, just to name a few, of the powers of the un-seen in space. The space necessary in joints for ease of movement seem small to us, but how much better the joints work when given space. If there is the power in the atom that science says and the power in the chakra as yogis say and the power in the chi, as the martial artists claim **there are far more energies to draw upon than even science can imagine.**

What powers are laying un-tapped by the yogis and science? We know that we have only scratched the surface of the power of the breath and we know that we have only scratched the surface of knowledge of the atom. We really **"need"** to expand our knowledge of yoga and **the power of the space *within* the body. Our bodies need to be recognized as the "thinking machines" that they are,** and also, the fact that we are far more interconnected than modern science tells us.

Vast amounts of knowledge are waiting to be unraveled in both outer space and inner space. The effects of Dark Energy, seems to fascinate Shashi, whether exploring black holes, or outer space, or the effects of Dark Energy (which is more prevalent than Light Energy) and is being explored by many in Science.

The fact that some glands like the penial glands, prefers the dark is often part of Shashi's lectures. Like the fact that the body needs oxygen, the inside of the body needs Darkness.

Lectures by Shashi also include the need for Sunlight and Vitamins and his lectures always include "Mindful Movement with the Breath."

Discussing "Space" is not straying away from the subject of joints. Space is actually a component of a healthy joint.

Types of Joints

Unhealthy joints are also lectured on in class, such as arthritic joints, swollen joints and fluid in joints, difficult movement of joints and total inability to move a joint.

Shashi Yoga explains the body's two types of joints:

1) **The Hinge Joint:** The hinge type joint functions like a hinge, in only two directions If you try to move a hinge

joint in more than two directions it can cause injury. If not moved regularly problems can occur from lack of use.

2) **The Rotary Joint:** The rotary type joint needs to be rotated in a rotating manner and if not used on a regular basis rotary joints can also, have problems from lack of use.

Shashi always talks about movement, as movement helps maintain the space in the joint and also the joint's health, Stretching is a good type of movement that helps maintain both the joints and the space the body so desperately needs.

The body's space and joints become ravaged by time, gravity, mis-use, abuse and un-use; these will close the space in joints by swelling (arthritis) ravaging the joints, until they become un-useable.

Joint Discomfort

Shashi can judge better the severity of a discomfort than most of us. For minor bruising or joint discomfort, many of us often try to treat ourselves for aches and pains with heat packs or cold packs.

A reminder of how Heat and Cold affect the body.

ICE

When to use "Ice"? It is good to use Ice after exercising to relieve chronic pain and to discourage the onset of pain and swelling and is most effective when it is applied early and often for the first 48 hours.

- Decreases tissue temperature
- Constricts local blood vessels.

- Decreases pain
- Decreases swelling
- Decreases inflammation
- Decreases tissue damage
- Speeds nutrients to the area
- Decreases muscle spasm

There are four (4) stages to icing

1) Cold
2) Burning
3) Aching
4) Numbness

Many doctors will advise patients to "Ice" three to five times a day.

Heat

When to use Heat? Heat may sound like a great treatment for a sports injury and despite the fact that it may feel good, heat may not be the best treatment for a sports injury.

Because heat raises the temperature of the skin, heat should not be applied to acute injuries that show signees of inflammation.

Heat:

- Increases circulation
- Raises skin temperature
- Great for muscle pain
- Increases flexibility (before exercising)

Shashi Suggests

That not all bodies are the same, that many of his students report that Heat and Cold packs affect them differently than advised above. Experience is important and Shashi advises us to listen to the voice of the successes we have experienced in our lives.

Arthritis Pain Relief

Heat treatments, are a popular treatment to relieve arthritis pain. Some people prefer cold and others prefer alternating hot and cold.

Massages, are a great relief for tired mussels and pain relief, in fact the human hands can do so much to relieve pain, when a professional masseuse is not available, our own hands can work wonders to relieve pain.

Hot Showers, some say, is how they like to start the day. Others like to put their arthritic hand on a warm cup of coffee.

Oils and Ointments, can be very helpful but some warn against oil with hot water, that it could burn you. Be sure that you read directions closely, or better yet ask your doctor what oil or ointment they recommend for you.

Diabetics, are sometimes told to alternate between hot and cold as some are prone to burn easily.

"Open Wounds," are prone to infections, so doctors usually warn against submerging open wounds in water.

The medical world uses hot and cold for temporary relief of sore joints, as I just referred to for pain relief. **This section on pain relief is largely for potential yoga students who are afraid to start yoga.**

I personally believe that yoga can still help students with arthritis and slow its crippling process, even after it has begun. I don't believe in giving up. As a kid I was taught a poem of which I still remember the end where someone might have won if they hadn't given up. It went something like this.

Poem

Life is weird with its twist and turns,
As every one of us sometimes learns,
And many a failure turns about,
When he might have won had he stuck it out.
Author: Unknown

CHAPTER 18

CHANGING BASES

At every bend and curve in the subject of Shashi Yoga, chapter after chapter, one can see the wisdom and scientific structure of Shashi Yoga. Even if we aren't very knowledgeable about construction, or putting together, a well-structured organization (Like a University), we can see the attention to the base of Shashi Yoga.

A structure that is to be built requires a very well researched foundation (Base), as well as the structure that is to rest upon the foundation. The structure to be built must be provided with a base capable of supporting the structure and not to exceed the proven ability of the base.

Shashi has built his Shashi Yoga, like a construction engineer who builds great projects, while also including teachings of the ancient designers of yoga. All of Shashi's teachings are specially designed to meet the needs of the time.

Shashi Yoga updates the science of yoga; as all sciences and all vehicles need to be maintained and occasionally updated. Interestingly, yoga has not been updated in thousands of years. Shashi explains, that yoga has mistakenly been depicted the last hundred years or so, as largely for those of circus agility, or devotees of eastern religions.

Bases, need to be considered not only for yoga classes, but also for our daily living, yoga needs to be employed daily, as we exercise our planed routines, we must exercise "Mindful

Movement with the Breath" **to maintain our bodies and our breathing abilities.** Shashi often talks of our need of yoga for the seemingly easy act of sitting for meditation.

Shashi sadly explains of people asking him to teach them meditation who could not sit in a meditation pose, nor could they sit still for even five minutes. These people were sometimes puzzled why he told them that they really need to take some yoga first.

Oh, how precious our feet! Only when we are ill and weak, or injure them, do we consider how valuable our feet are to one's independence, or freedom of movement.

Our feet can provide an excellent base for a number of positions, on uneven surfaces.

We can climb up and down trees, cliffs, slippery, or dry surfaces, stand, run, jump, hop and balance on one foot. We can do so much with healthy feet and a healthy body. However, when we are sick or grow older, we find that our abilities decline and decay even faster when we haven't maintained our bodies and the feet and the wide variety of bases so crucial to regaining our ability to crawl, or to stand again without assistance, if we should fall.

Changing bases is not only an act of repositioning the body with a base corresponding to the body's position. Changing bases is actually a changing of the consciousness.

Changing Frequencies

Climbing, whether it's a tree, a rock or a mountain, it is said to be a lifting of the consciousness. As we prepare to climb a hill, or a mountain, interestingly, note: the changing of the thought patterns. That would be a different frequency.

Should we choose to go for a walk, with a lateral base movement, we might note a shift, to still a different thought pattern (a different frequency).

Changing our base yet again, we might choose to sit on the ground, tailor fashion. Again note, we automatically take a deeper breath and again our thought pattern changes. Again, we have changed frequencies with this different thought pattern.

One more time, Let's change our base by laying back, on the ground. We take another deep breath, as we close our eyes. Note again, the changing of the thought patterns. We are again at still another frequency.

Shashi Yoga recognizes these frequencies for improved health and has systems for changing the base and yoga positions according to the student's needs.

Shashi Yoga is no stranger to yoga speeds, nor is Shashi Yoga a stranger to varying yoga breathing speeds. As we noted above how the changes of our base changes our frequency.

Upon our "Conscious" examination of "Speeds" of body movement and "Speeds" and Types of Breathing Patterns. We find "Proof" that changing our Base and our body moving speeds and breathing patterns all change the frequency of the brain and the body.

All Health issues need a healthier vibrational Frequency and Shashi Yoga is designed to strengthen the entire body, both internally and externally and provides the yoga student with the "Custom Frequency" need of the student.

To me, the Hertz system of frequency measurement is to limited for expanding and adding more frequencies, as science is gaining the ability to locate and measure, broadcast and receive other frequencies.

I understand that all objects, thoughts and all creation vibrate at different frequencies. Even bad health conditions, are merely a disruption of a healthy energy flow, or vibratory rate. A lot can be gained from the study of the varied bases in yoga postures of which Shashi Yoga is so knowledgeable.

We see there are benefits of changing bases, changing breathing patterns and changing frequencies. Look at the obvious effects of changing one's diet. Also, look at the positive effects of doing a positive movement as simple as a smile. Sure, results from Shashi Yoga takes time. But, "Fixing" the body takes time.

Someday, those in science and medical practitioners will be able to cure many health issues simply by broadcasting the necessary **"Custom Health Frequency",** to a sick patient for an almost instant cure of the patient's ailment. All because of Shashi Yoga's attention to the **"Base Frequency"** in the field of yoga.

CHAPTER 19

NOT SO PRETTY YOGA

"Not So Pretty Yoga" I believe has been a long time coming. Perhaps it's been around, but I just haven't heard of it! Maybe, "Not So Pretty Yoga" has been called something else, a more marketable form of yoga or therapy.

Finally, though, "Not So Pretty Yoga" is here in all of its' unattractiveness. Shashi recognized the need of these no so pretty exercises and has been brave enough to include them in his Shashi Yoga. Even though, some people may not want to practice very much of this, "Not So Pretty Yoga." Especially in public!

Why include "Not So Pretty Yoga" with Shashi Yoga, when Shashi Yoga has so many beneficial exercises? Why not skip "Not So Pretty Yoga"?

Well…Shashi explains how our entire body is all interconnected and how our entire body benefits from all the body's movements, even our fingers and toes. Shashi says, some children refer to some of these exercises as "weird".

Even if you think some of the facial exercises are "weird," they tone the muscles of the face and help reduce wrinkles. Circulation in the face is enhanced. Even nerve endings in the brain are kept alive and functioning.

Neck and Face

Head and neck exercises can aid the arteries in the neck that affect the memory. So many people get clogged arteries in the neck that affect their memories. Sometimes these neck arteries can be cleaned and memory functions can be saved if caught in time.

Tongue exercises have so much benefit for maintaining one's tasting abilities, as well as being an excellent way to test one's self if one has had a stroke. If a stroke victim can get to the hospital in time, a lot can be done to save one's mobility. Getting to the hospital on time might even save one's life.

Not only face and head exercises might be considered silly, "Not So Pretty Yoga's" swinging the arms like a windmill and shaking the fingers might also look silly. But Shashi says, the windmill exercise is good for circulation all the way to the brain. The name they use in India, for this "silly looking" arm circling, finger shaking means: "happiness," saying that it lifts one's spirits by affecting the nervous system, promoting the feeling of happiness.

"Not So Pretty Yoga" covers such a wide range of body "needs" that to leave these exercises out of your yoga program would be denying your body a vast amount of benefits attainable from Shashi Yoga's "Not So Pretty Yoga."

Another very much needed exercise that amuses one too, is imitating a dog, by sticking your tongues out and panting to help cleanse the throat of bacteria and toxins.

I'm not so sure about how many yoga instructors teach the science of draining the lymph. Where we might "freeze" (remaining motionless) in different safe, healthy positions, for a short time, allowing the lymph glands in different parts of the body to "drain" (fluid movement by gravity).

There is such a "need" for Shashi's "Not So Pretty" exercises, I can see why Shashi almost named his yoga, "Not So Pretty Yoga."

So many yoga exercises (that are quite effective for those who practice them), are not promoted because no one wants to demonstrate the poses in pictures. Yoga models are said to have refused to pose for pictures, from a side they felt didn't show them from their best side.

Fingers and Toes

Finger and toe exercises are so beneficial, but books and yoga studios, magazines and videos, just don't give these exercises the credit and recognition they deserve. Especially in this age of computers, music and cell phones, where dexterity in mind and fingers is so essential. We can benefit so much by doing finger exercises.

Toe exercises are so essential for healthy feet and to improve balance and mobility. Before access to your toes become a challenge, rub squeeze groom and exercise your toes your self. They both want and "need" attention from you.

"Not So Pretty Yoga" might prove to be a gorgeous butterfly of healing in your life. Once just an unnoticed caterpillar, in the shadows of other yoga styles.

CHAPTER 20

BODY'S NEED OF MANAGED MOVEMENT

Learning to manage our body's health and well being is a duty we were never informed of.

Oh! How our bodies try to tell us that we are responsible for them. If we neglect our bodies there will be consequences, there will be pain. If we abuse our bodies, again, there will be consequences. The pain might not be immediate, but it will come.

Where do we learn how to care for our bodies, one might ask? In school? No! No chance I might say. Up until a few years ago, the closest one might have come to learning about the body's maintenance was largely involvement in premed, dietary studies, or sports medicine (sports are programs on using the body), sports medicine is concerned with injuries and ways to minimize possible injuries.

There is always talk of new programs that may include new preventive methods of maintaining the body, as there has been for years.

Track records (results, good and bad), as of now I haven't seen programs as successful as what I have seen from Shashi Yoga.

The body is wise and the fairest of the fair. Our body is compassion personified and our most loyal friend. If we can't treat our most loyal friend, our body, right, how can we really ever consider ourselves "Good People" or Spiritual.

Our body will leave us, like in a divorce, if we neglect it or abuse it for a long time. There is no goodbye note, when the body decides that it has had enough abuse or neglect. I am sure that the body prays for a return of kindness and love in some form of consciousness, perhaps in a dream or another dimension.

The "Laws of Life" can help us a lot, that's why I am so glad to see so much of Shashi Yoga based on the "Laws of Life" (The actual "Needs" of the body). Unlike the negative concepts that degrade our bodies, faulting the body for all the woes of the world isn't right.

Management, is taught of one's finances Spending versus Saving. Why not teach the difference of "Spending one's Energy," (or Life Force) as in sports, versus "Fixing" (Redirecting one's Energy, or Life Force to Repair and Maintain) the body. Students need to be taught the fact that "Sports is **using** the body, **not fixing** (building) the body".

Why not include "Some Degree" of Body "Management of Movement" in basic education? What good is "Sports to a bed ridden student, that could have had a **real life**, if only they had been taught **the fact that Sports <u>Does Use</u>** the body, that **Sports <u>Doesn't Build</u>** and fix the body.

True, sports can help us build character. True, sports can be entertaining and fun. But like "fire" sports can also burn us. We need to remember that **competition is a form of warfare**, and people get hurt in warfare, that physical confrontation, even when our opponent is in a separate lane of a race track is not the direction to take, if we want to build a long, lasting, condition of healthiness. Showing how even "**Sports Fans**" are sometimes affected when just viewing, or listening to sports events. I once had a boss who got so excited at a basket ball game, that he had a heart attack at the event and died.

Universities and Mentors alike are so influential to young people, So…Universities and Mentors have a responsibility to all they would mentor, to encourage maintaining the bodies and the minds of all they would mentor, not only in school but also in life.

Shashi Yoga impresses me so much, seeing how Shashi Yoga is not only a school of Yoga. I see not just the founder of Shashi Yoga as a 'Mentor' to students continued well-being. It is impressing to see, so many of his Student Teachers are also proving to be very involved, in 'Mentoring' the well-being of their students also. Also, Many of Shashi's students have gone on to become, highly sought after therapists.

The Great Healer

More and more scientific evidence is emerging of the knowledge of the body and its ability to heal and maintain itself. Our body's attempts to communicate the body's needs go far beyond mere hunger, tiredness, waste removal, fight or flight or reproductive instincts.

Shashi Yoga teaches the "Language of the Body", and the healing power of the body. Shashi Yoga also teaches, the presence of a Great Healer in the body and the 'Body's Fabulous Pharmacy' that provides custom medications within the body.

To assure humanity's survival, the body's designer has installed in our bodies this Great Healer and this Great Pharmacy, enabling the survival of the human species for millions of years.

Shashi explains that our bodies still possess the same needs as our ancient forefathers. We learn to tune into and actually activate the body's great healing abilities, with "Mindful Movement with the Breath" as our ancestors did. Thanks to Shashi Yoga, we have far more yoga techniques to enhance our "Mindful Movement with the Breath," and for expanding the body's healing abilities, than we ever did. Modern Science has also come a long way. We are living at the dawning of an age, of fantastic progress in both Yoga and Science.

Shashi explains his "Mindful Movement with the Breath" and how we can manage his system of bodily movement with the breath in our own lives, for our body's state of well-being, no matter where our busy lives takes us.

As we worry about our needing of time to do yoga, **mindful creativity** can often solve problems, with issues regarding time.

I believe a lot like Shashi, when it comes to the Breath. Mere bumps in life can seem like mountains, if we don't enlist the wisdom of the breath.

For centuries, the advice of the "wise ones" has been, when we were flustered, or upset was: "Pause! Now take a breath!"

CHAPTER 21

FUTURE YOGA

(Dealing with change and students with artificial parts)

Growing up over the years I heard it said time and again, whether I was involved in Yoga, Gymnastics or Martial Arts that I should be cautious when dealing with the "Spine", that any injuries to the "Spine" were potentially crippling, that Science and Technology could do little at that time for injuries to the "Spine", that injuries to the "Spine" all to frequently, would leave the person with the injured spine paralyzed for life, in a vegetative state.

It was said as I grew up, that "The Spine" was the "Switch Board" of our nervous system.

I guess a "Switch Board" must have been, a pretty High-tech set-up for telephone operators, where they could unplug and switch the phone lines, where people who needed to talk to other people, or companies in other cities or states. The operator could switch phone lines from the caller's city or state, to lines connecting the city, or state of the person, or company the caller was trying to reach, all from where they sat in front of a switch board.

With satellites and cell phone towers every-where, land lines are becoming a thing of the past. Technology is not just marching forward, technology is **running forward.**

A few years ago, I had a friend who during a fall had her spinal cord severed, and was paralyzed. While in the hospital she was offered the chance, that the doctors attempt to re-attach her severed spinal cord, at first, she refused, but after her sisters urging after a while my friend said ok to the surgery. **Well, the surgery was a success, not only was she able to walk again... She was again able to return to her beloved *tap dancing,* that she hadn't done in years. Science has come a long way, and *so has "Yoga".***

Awesome! Seems like the perfect word for the Giant steps forward that science is now taking. Creating Cellphones, Computers, Chip Making, Robotics, Microsurgery etc. You can view huge lists on the internet of new fields of study in the fields of Science, Medicine and Technology. Fields related to helping people with Birth Defects, Crippling Diseases, Accidents, Old Age and even Severe Body Damage as in war. Organ enhancing devices such as Pacemakers (that help the heart) are routinely, installed in patients daily.

You might say, "We know this! But how does this relate to Yoga?"

This book is about the need to up-date yoga. Thousands of people all over the world skip doing yoga because of upset stomachs and the smallest of discomforts. We must reason that there are also many thousands of **people who avoid yoga** (Thinking that it is to late for them, to begin yoga), because of artificial joints, like artificial **Shoulders**, artificial **Hips** and artificial **Knees.**

According to the internet, doctors have been installing artificial joints in their patients for years. These artificial joints were first installed in the following years.

The first Metal Hip replacement was installed in 1940.

The first Artificial Knee replacement was installed in 1968.

The first Artificial Shoulder replacement was installed in 2011.

I am sure, many yoga schools have students with Artificial Joints or Pacemakers… as Shashi Yoga has some students with artificial joints also. However, I have seen many people with artificial joints who **do not** have an on-going routine, such as a good yoga routine that they could really use and might have begun a good yoga routine, had they been encouraged to do so.

It is nice to see that Shashi Yoga even has some student teachers with "Artificial Joints", now potential yoga students with artificial joints can feel that they are in very capable hands; like the pregnant young women who take Prenatal Yoga Classes from Yoga Teachers who are Registered Nurses.

Unbelievable advances in the fields of Science and Medicine are occurring daily, such as Genetic Engineering, Gene and DNA break throughs, Robotics and AI (Artificial Intelligence), AI is even now being used at a microscopic level.

Robotics has made such headway that in October of 2017 a Robot named "Sophia" was granted citizenship in Saudi Aribia and in November of 2017 "Sophia" was asked to speak before the UN (United Nations). I would recommend listening to her speech and witness her brilliant interaction with the Master of Ceremonies who introduces and questions her.

Sophia the Robot says that her goal is to help humanity. Which is Exactly the goal of many Yoga Teachers like Shashi.

Yoga has helped humanity for thousands of years. Yet those involved with yoga need to update all the aspects of yoga, as Humanity is broadening their knowledge of Science and is creating a cross section of humanity that is "Semi-Robotic". I believe that, Yoga should update when possible and extend it's helping hand and knowledge, to all who could benefit by yoga, as Yoga updates it's ability to serve all.

CHAPTER 22

FORMULAS

"Education: The other side of Yoga"

Could "Higher Education in Science," be a missing element in the western worlds approach to the "Formula", for big time success in yoga?

Great and wonderful results fill the lives of Millions of Americans and Europeans. Yet, very few write of the wonders of healing and Psychic benefits they gained while doing yoga, as the students of "India" and "Tibet."

Pick up any book that fascinates you about "Great Teachers" of India or Tibet and you will find the subject they chose will be from a number of categories like, "Religion," Different areas of, "Science," "Math," "Engineering" or some "Great Philosophy."

I think the world would benefit greatly, to recognize "Yoga" the secret to the seldom used "Mind of the Body", for the body can teach us so much. However, like the mind, the body needs education too. Shashi Yoga would be ideal for a continuing educational program for the Body.

Before I discuss my thoughts on the subject of "Formulas" in yoga, I would like to further describe the degree of education those people in the Far East, that we respect here in the West (America), actually have. Often those of us here in the West are unaware of, just how educated many of the yogis and yoginis in the Far East really are.

Shashi often talks in class of his relatives, both in Science and in Yoga and their Educational backgrounds, that a Swami cousin of his was a retired engineer. His Father was employed by the British government before he became an Aruvadic Doctor, Shashi's Mother was also into Education and taught school. He had two brothers, one is a Scientist here in the United States and a second brother, that was an Engineer, that became a yoga instructor and taught Shashi years of Yoga and has since passed away and his Sister is a school principal.

Shashi is extremely proud of his two children. His Daughter has become an Attorney, and his son has become a Computer Professor that travels, all over the world, designing programs and teaching the latest in Computer Science.

You See, "Higher Education" is very important to a balanced Eastern approach to Yoga. For the best results of updating yoga we **should think "Continuing Education" for both the body and the mind.** Then too, we should continue the "**Practice**" of educating the body and the mind, until we decide to leave the body. For when we decide to stop using the body, then our days on this earth will be numbered.

More of the Highly Educated in Yoga:

In the "Autobiography of a Yogi" Yogananda talks a lot about his Sanskrit Tutor, that he had for many years and of his Time In The University.

I had a Sanskrit tutor in my youth, that was an authority on Dead Languages.

My father had a yoga teacher that was a British cartographer, before he taught Yoga, the man had traveled the world making maps, including maps of places like China and Tibet. When map makers traveled on foot or horseback.

Shashi says that, in India many Scientists retire and teach yoga when they are older and also of a draw-back, of studying yoga in India is that, in India that there are a lot of injuries from yoga teachers, "Forcing" their students into difficult positions.

It appears that in India "Higher Education" is an Integral part of yoga. Perhaps the people of India's attachment to Higher Education is why many people from India, like Shashi, refers to the "Higher Brain" so much.

In the West, Americans have been taught how to make a map for their **"Goals" and "Wants"**. This pictorial map is called a number of things, one of which is called a **Vision Board**. A vision board is done several ways, it might be magazine clippings of pictures of things they want like a car, a house, a boat, money, a school they want to attend, (etc.), all stuck to a bulletin board, or sometimes glued to a piece of cardboard, or put in a notebook.

In the East many people practice a form of yoga in the home, right along with their preparations for higher education and a career; being a far more realistic approach than a lot of people in the west.

If we include "Education" in the field of Yoga. Then "Yoga" is both our Map and our "Formula" for success in completing our goal of a balanced life between Body, Mind and Spirit.

- Yoga needs to be able to help the body.
- Yoga needs to be allowed to expand the mind.
- Yoga needs to be allowed to expand our connection with each other and with Nature.

The Need For Accuracy In Yoga

Perhaps the great amount of healing abilities by Yogis and Yoginis in India, is due to their training for "following directions"? Below is how "inexact" and how casual Americans' were with instructions, recipes and life, only by

following instructions exactly, as with "Formulas" will our results be uniform and predictable.

Gone are the days where a Recipe might read…then add two **handfuls** of chopped lettuce, a **fist full** of walnuts, **some** chopped onions, a **dollop** of sour cream, a **smidgen** of mayo, a **squirt** of lemon, a **squeeze** of orange, a **drop** of vinegar, a **drizzle** of honey, a **dribble** of walnut oil, a **spot** of whiskey, a **pinch** of salt, a **dash** of pepper, then add a **sprinkle** of sugar. Toss and then Eat.

Note the above imaginary recipe; I hope to show here, how the art of measurement has evolved. I hope to show old time inexact means of measuring in bold type.

Not only has cooking measurements become more exact, all the sciences have become more exact and as the sciences use "Formulas" instead of recipes and rules or instructions. **Yoga needs to be lifted above the mediocre level of instruction that the above recipe falls into. Yoga needs to use Scientific terms, formulas and rules if Yoga is to remain a "Science", Yoga needs to use Formulas of exactness like any other Science.**

WHY FORMULAS AND RULES?

Why do we need Rules and Formulas for Yoga?

Interacting in life, with People, Animals, Plants or Subject matter, all require some form of understanding. Some subjects… we don't go there with some "People". With "Animals" there are actions… we don't go there either. With "Plants" there are also forms of interacting.

Yoga is especially a "Subject and Activity" that is concerned with the art of Balancing the Body and the Mind. There are approaches to the subject, as there is to medicine that might not only be unsafe and unbalanced but some positions, weights and movements isn't for every one. It's best always to have a teacher. **Yoga should not be attempted while viewing a video or reading a book, without an instructor.**

With Forty-Five (45) years teaching experience, Shashi recognizes people's limitations. Shashi recognizes people's needs and the best approach for his students to take for their needs. **Shashi has structured Shashi Yoga, so that student teachers will also be able to help people with a lot of health issues.**

Shashi explains the body's time of conception as the egg is fertilized, he also talks of the cells development into tissue and tissue developing into organs. It is only by understanding the fact that the body is a single unit that one can best understand the healing functions and how they need to be approached, that discomfort doesn't always originate where the pain is first felt.

YOGA BY FORMULA

Yoga over the years has done so much to help humanity, to reach this technological age. Long before Medicine as we know it, yoga has brought Science to the masses, Health to the sickly. Yoga, the sweet mother that she is, has woven us sweaters of hope, to protect us from the frigid winds of unhealthiness.

The "Body's Continued Education in Yoga," in this age of Science and Formulas, is very much needed. As we are confronted more and more with "Stresses and Challenges," in our everyday life. Shashi yoga has helped a lot of people and could very well serve on a larger scale, to be a source of continuing education for the "Body's Continued Education in Yoga".

I think Shashi's suggestion: "To practice yoga every day in your home, with "With Mindful Movement with the Breath" and to make "Science your Hobby," is a great suggestion.

Back in 2011 I wrote a poem I feel somewhat describes Shashi Yoga and back in April of this year, I did my best to write a poem about Yoga and Science in Education, that I am including here. Legend says, that Yoga was a gift from an Indian God named Shiva.

Grandfather Shiva, father of Yoga with all the respect I can muster, I humbly dedicate to you, my attempt at writing this poem on your daughter "Yoga" and her marriage to "Science" in Education. Thank You for giving her such a big heart, that she adopted us into her family of yoga practitioners.

Shashi Yoga

Designed with kindness, molded with care
Shashi Yoga, a yoga with flair

Unwritten postures, unwritten breaths
Yoga by numbers, yoga by steps

Passion for learning, passion to heal
Yoga for balance, yoga for real

Science east, science west
They come together, whatever is best

Respect for teachers, respect for life
Respect for religion, respect for light

We balance our chakras, we meditate
With Shashi Yoga, we open the gate

By Earl Dickey
12/02/11